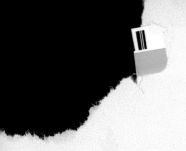

Also by Claire McCarthy, M.D.

Learning How the Heart Beats

Everyone's Children

A Pediatrician's Story of an Inner-City Practice

Claire McCarthy, M.D.

SCRIBNER

SCRIBNER
Rockefeller Center
1230 Avenue of the Americas
New York, NY 10020

Designed by Colin Joh
Text in Bembo

Manufactured in the United States of America

10 9 8 7 6 5 4 3 2 1

Library of Congress Cataloging-In-Publication Data

Library of Congress Cataloging-in-Publication Data
McCarthy, Claire, M.D.
Everyone's children: a pediatrician's story of
An inner-city practice/by Claire McCarthy.
p. cm.
1. McCarthy, Claire, M.D.
2. Pediatricians—Massachusetts—Boston—Biography.
3. Martha Eliot Health Center. I. Title.
RJ43.M33A3   1998
618.92'0009—dc21
[B] 97-28289
CIP

ISBN 978-0-743-24268-4

For information regarding the special discounts for bulk purchases, please contact Simon &
Schuster Special Sales at 1-800-456-6798 or business@simonandschuster.com

For Aidan, my angel,
and for Evelyn Boyle McCarthy,
who holds him tight for me in Heaven

Acknowledgments

I would like to thank Jane Rosenman, my editor at Scribner, for her encouragement and her insightful editing. I would also like to thank Margot Rohrer and Karen Darcy for their invaluable perspective and guidance. My literary agent, Doe Coover, was helpful with many aspects of this book; I appreciate her input and her friendship. And I am grateful to Mark Brown, my husband and *compañero*, for his patience and support.

Most of all, I would like to thank the staff and patients of Martha Eliot Health Center. It is an honor to work with them and for them.

The characters in this book are based on real people and their experiences, but names and identifying details have been changed to protect their privacy.

Everyone's Children

One

They came in by themselves—three teenage boys, dazed and bleeding, at lunchtime. The security guard brought them to Pediatrics. We were on the first floor, close to the front door, so we got all the emergencies, whether they were pediatric emergencies or not.

I was the only one there; everyone else had gone out for lunch. I led them into Room Two and sat them down, one on the exam table and the others in two chairs I brought in. All three were African-American, and all three were dressed in the uniform of the housing developments: oversized T-shirts, baggy and drooping jeans, high-top sneakers. At night when I left the clinic I'd see groups of boys dressed this way, walking confidently through the housing development. Some seemed very young; none of them looked older than twenty-five. They were mostly African-American or Latino. I never looked at them very long, of course. I didn't dare. I knew that many carried weapons, and I knew that some of them used them. I was an unlikely target—they were much more likely to hurt one another or someone from a different gang—but I didn't want to take any chances. I did my best to slip by unnoticed.

But here, in Room Two, they weren't threatening. They'd come for help. I put on gloves and began to examine them. As I did, I asked what had happened.

They were on the subway, one of them told me, and were attacked by "some guys" with knives and a board. The boys got off at the Jackson Square stop and ran into the housing development. They didn't know if they were followed. They didn't look back.

All three had scratches and bruises. The biggest one, whom I had directed to the exam table, had a bad bump on his head from the board. It was bleeding, but didn't need stitches. He looked like he felt dizzy; I had him lie down. His heart rate and blood pressure were normal, and his pupils were of equal size and reacted normally to light. I didn't think the injury was serious, but the lump on the side of his head was quite large. He was going to need observation, and possibly some X rays of his skull. The other two had bad gashes, one on his left hand and the other on the back of his arm; they were deep, and were going to need lots of careful stitching, more than I could manage at the clinic. I decided to send them all to the emergency room at Children's Hospital.

"I'm going to get you guys cleaned up and bandaged, and then I'm going to get an ambulance to take you over to the emergency room," I said. I got their names and birth dates, so that I could call the record room for their charts. The big one and the one with the cut hand were sixteen; the other was fourteen.

"Do you know who the guys that attacked you were, or why they attacked you?" I asked. They shook their heads. I didn't believe them.

"Did this have to do with gang stuff?" I asked. The sixteen-year-olds looked away and down, not responding. The fourteen-year-old nodded, almost imperceptibly.

I cleaned them up with Betadine and water and gauzes, one at a time. I did it as gently as I could, for they winced and tried to pull away from me. The sixteen-year-old with the cut hand cried. The big one looked like he wanted to. The fourteen-year-old looked at me with big eyes and asked me if he was cut real bad.

"Yes," I said. "But you're going to be okay, don't worry."

They were quiet and shaky, like little children. They seemed comforted when I taped bandages across their wounds, comforted to have them covered, and it almost seemed like they leaned in to me slightly as I finished taping, as if seeking to be held. I wanted to hold them, actually; in that moment it felt as if that was what they needed most of all. The air in the room was filled with their vulnerability and fear.

There was a knock on the door; it was Rick, one of the youth outreach workers. He'd heard what happened from some kids in the housing development. He asked if he could talk to the boys.

"Sure," I said. "I need to go call the ambulance and their parents anyway."

At the mention of parents the fourteen-year-old looked startled. The sixteen-year-olds didn't respond. I shut the door behind me.

I called for the ambulance, and then went through the boys' charts and found phone numbers. Nobody answered at the numbers for the sixteen-year-olds. A woman answered at the fourteen-year-old's number; her voice was slurred and loud and she said that it served him right. I asked her if she would go meet him at the emergency room. "Maybe," she said, and hung up.

I saw the ambulance arriving. I knocked softly on the door of Room Two and went in. Rick was talking.

"This is what I was trying to tell you the other night," he was saying. "One of you is going to end up dead next time. This has got to stop."

Everything felt different in the room. The big one on the exam table had sat up. He leaned against the wall, a little unsteadily but with determination. The other two were slouched in their chairs, no longer shaky. They didn't look at Rick. Their faces had taken on that purposeful blankness that was so familiar to me; this is how they looked outside, in the housing development. The air was no longer filled with vulnerability and fear. Whatever had been opened was shut.

Things are opened, sometimes, at the clinic. Not always, and usually not for very long, but sometimes one catches a glimpse of what is underneath and possible. Those glimpses, I think, are part of what keeps me going.

★ ★ ★

We actually don't see many stabbings or shootings or things like that in the clinic. Most of what we see is fairly routine medicine: things like colds, ear infections, asthma, minor injuries, school physicals—the same as any other pediatric practice sees. And most of the people who come to the clinic are law-abiding, not drug addicted, and take good care of themselves and their children. But we are in an inner-city housing development, which like any other has its share of poverty, drugs, and violence. Unexpected things can happen. One needs to be prepared.

The clinic is called Martha Eliot Health Center and it is in the Bromley-Heath Housing Development, in Jamaica Plain, a community of Boston. In 1996 a new building for the clinic was built, on the edge of the housing development near Centre Street, but the building I went to work at in the summer of 1991 was an old, squat brick building like most of the others around it. There are some high-rises in the housing development too, also brick, rising up tall and stark. The Boston Housing Authority has been fixing things up, renovating and planting. There is still a lot of dirt and cracked cement, but in certain pockets and places it is pretty—another glimpse of what is underneath and possible.

The clinic was born of the efforts of the residents of Bromley-Heath to bring health services into their community. It started out as a storefront maternal-child health service funded by the Office of Economic Opportunity and operated under the license of Children's Hospital of Boston and the Peter Bent Brigham Hospital (which went on to become part of what is now Brigham and Women's Hospital). In 1973 Children's Hospital took over the clinic operation. Along with pediatrics, the clinic offers adult medicine, obstetrics and gynecology, mental health services, nutrition counseling, dental services, and optometry. There are also outreach programs and a program for HIV testing and counseling, as well as a substance abuse treatment program. It is constantly losing money, as nearly two-thirds of the patients have no insurance. Most of the rest are on Medicaid.

Three-quarters of the patients are Spanish-speaking. This in part reflects the community; although the people of the housing development are mostly African-American, this area of Jamaica Plain is very Latino, with some census tracts that are almost entirely Latino. But patients come from other communities too, either because they used to live in Jamaica Plain and they don't want to change health-care providers, or because they hear that we offer services in both Spanish and English. Many of our patients are recent immigrants who do not speak any English, and many of them are undocumented.

As soon as one walks into the clinic, one hears Spanish. The patients are speaking it, and as many of the staff are Latino the casual banter between the staff is as likely to be in Spanish as in English. All the signs are in both languages. It is almost like being in a different country.

It *is* a different country. It is different from anywhere I have ever been or lived. There are different customs, there are different laws; the justice is different and the possibilities are different too. The language is different, even when I'm speaking English, for words have different meanings there. It took me a long time to understand this. It took me a long time to see that I had to start at the beginning, at the bottom, and learn things from there.

Where I come from is a different country, too: that part, or that type, of America where money is not a problem and education, including higher education, is taken for granted. My mother is a lawyer and my father a history professor. We lived in nice suburbs with good public schools, and from an early age my sister and I were told that we should pursue not just a college education but a professional degree as well. We didn't question this. I went to Princeton, and then to Harvard Medical School. This life, this country, seemed normal and routine. It was all I knew; it was how everybody I knew lived.

Not far from the clinic there are mansions. They are around Jamaica Pond, a lovely pond with a gracious, clean park surrounding it and an elegant boathouse. The neighborhood there is affluent and beautiful; the houses have landscaped backyards and there are expensive cars parked in the driveways.

The Harvard Medical Area is close to the clinic, too, perhaps a twenty-minute walk. The medical school is there, along with four major teaching hospitals, and laboratories filled with eminent researchers. People come from all over the world for the very latest in medical treatments, or to study and take part in research. When you walk the sidewalks there, it is like being in a magical kingdom. Important things happen here, the buildings seem to say, Miracles happen here.

And yet steps away from the pond and the medical area, at the clinic, there is no affluence and there are very few miracles. Steps away, the world is impossibly different. These kinds of contrasts are actually very common; all around the world poor is pushed up next to rich, cultures very distinct live back-to-back. But rarely is there mixing, or blurring of boundaries. With few exceptions, people keep within the confines of where they've been and what they know.

Not that I blame them, really. Crossing, or even just blurring, boundaries is hard. I am a different woman than I was in the summer of 1991. The world has changed for me, irrevocably. I cannot go back to the country I came from—nor can I live in this new one. I am in between.

There was an iron fence across the front of the original Martha Eliot Clinic, and two sets of doors going in, which gave the security guard a chance to assess who was coming in before they were actually in. The lobby was the only bright and cheery part of the clinic. There were big windows, and a high ceiling with a skylight. A colorful rug covered the floor, and there was a small plastic slide and a few other large, durable toys. Because Pediatrics was right off the lobby, the lobby was usually full of children and their noise. They ran between the chairs, chasing each other; they laughed, they sang, they cried. The mothers sat in the chairs, holding the infants and the ones who were too sick and miserable to play, watching the other children, talking to the other mothers. There were fathers, too, but mostly there were mothers. Most of the families who come to Pediatrics are headed by single mothers.

My days at the clinic are filled with mothers and children. I spend my days talking to them, about everything from coughs to school problems to favorite cartoons. I am a mother too, so we share stories. We laugh and sometimes we cry together.

The voices of the mothers are always in my head. I hear them telling me about their lives, their worries, and their joys. When I close my eyes I see their faces, and the faces of the children, some of whom I have known since they were born. These people have become so important to me that it is hard to imagine working anywhere else.

There is a rawness that poverty brings to people and their lives, a shearing off of veneers. I see so much that is difficult and sad in my work, but I also get to see human resilience, strength, and beauty at their best. Life gets whittled down to what is crucial and simple. Small triumphs are huge. A kindness can mean everything.

There was a set of swinging doors that led off the lobby into Pediatrics. It wasn't much: a narrow corridor lined with the secretaries' area, a staff room, a med room (a room where medications and supplies were kept), and four examination rooms that led down to a very small internal waiting room. Off this waiting room, which we filled with donated toys and books that were frequently stolen, were three more exam rooms and the caseworkers' office.

The staff room was a cluttered, stuffy, small room with shelves, lockers, file cabinets, and narrow tables against the walls where the staff sat to do their paperwork. If you looked closely enough, you could usually find a cockroach. There was a microwave that the whole clinic used, and a small refrigerator where we stored our lunches. Sometimes we share our lunches with the patients. The children are often hungry.

The exam rooms varied in size, but none was very big. Despite the professional cleaning service that came every night, they were dingy. They needed painting, and the furniture was old and worn. Each room had a dented metal desk, an exam table, a sink, a scale, and a couple of unmatched chairs. On the wall over each exam table hung an otoscope, an ophthalmoscope, and an apparatus to measure blood pressure. There was an occasional old picture hung on the wall, but for the most part the walls were bare. Everything was minimal, somehow, at the clinic. Even in the new building, with the clean, bright walls and new furniture, it is still minimal.

Everything is minimal, but it never feels empty. It is always full of noise and motion. At times, it is absolute chaos. But even in the early morning, before the patients have come, it feels full. The rooms echo with voices. Stories linger in the air.

I hadn't planned on doing this kind of medicine when I started medical school. Not that I had another plan, because I didn't. I had decided when I was twelve that I wanted to be a doctor, and that's about as far as I took it. It wasn't until I actually got to medical school that I confronted the fact that I was going to have to make decisions about what kind of doctor I was going to be and where and how I was going to practice. So I watched the doctors around me, and tried on specialties like lab coats as I went through my rotations, seeing how they felt.

I discovered pretty quickly that I enjoyed spending time with patients much more than I enjoyed discussing cases and science with other doctors. Science was interesting to me, but not compelling—something I was terribly afraid to admit because science was what all conversations seemed to be centered upon. Spending time with patients was not consistently rewarded by the doctors who were training and evaluating me; finding the latest journal article on a particular illness or treatment was.

In pediatrics things were slightly better. The conversations still centered upon science, but there was also value placed on spending time with patients. I had always enjoyed being around children; I liked their optimism, their honesty, their playfulness. These qualities seemed to rub off a little on the pediatricians, who were in general more pleasant to be around than other kinds of doctors.

I did my pediatric residency training at Children's Hospital in Boston, a tertiary-care center affiliated with Harvard, which offers everything from transplants to baby shots, from the latest in chemotherapy to the latest in the treatment of behavioral problems. My three years there were an exhausting blur, working very long hours and straight through every third or fourth night. I worked on the wards, in the intensive care units, and in the emergency room. I did some outpatient medicine as well, rotating through the specialty clinics. One afternoon a week I saw patients for physicals and other routine appointments in the residents' clinic. One afternoon a week was frustratingly little to me, because it was the kind of medicine I was starting to like best.

I liked getting to know people and practicing medicine in the context of lives instead of the context of crises, as is so often the case in a tertiary-care setting. Primary care—going out and being a pediatrician instead of training in a subspecialty like pediatric cardiology—would allow me to do that. It made sense to me and for me. So did working at Martha Eliot.

I've made all of the major decisions in my life because they "made sense." It is a gut thing for me, making sense. It has to do with things feeling right, in an immediate, powerful, durable way. Choosing medicine felt that way. When I met my husband it felt that way, too; we were engaged less than six months later. It felt that way to go work at an inner-city clinic, although I couldn't explain it to anyone—and plenty of people wanted me to explain it. It was not exactly a common choice; of the fifteen or so senior residents in my class, only three of us went into primary care instead of subspecialties, and the other two who did primary care went to work in practices in wealthy suburbs of Boston. I wanted to go where I was needed and could possibly make a difference, that was certainly part of it. But there was something else, something that had to do with sorting out my life in general.

My life had always been defined by degrees, accomplishments, and income, by one's knowledge of literature, current events, the latest scientific achievement. The parameters were clear. It seemed like it should make sense, but I always had a nagging feeling that it didn't.

Later, after some time at the clinic, I realized that the reason my life didn't make sense was that it only made sense within its own paradigm. It only made sense to the people who belonged. I was looking for rules and reasons that would make sense no matter who one was or where one was. I was looking for things to define my life that would always and completely be right. I thought that I might be able to find them at the clinic.

I have certainly found extraordinary people there, staff and patients, people who are strong and brave and creative in ways I hope someday to be. I have met people who have survived, and are surviving, things I don't know if I could survive. I have learned much about being a mother, and have found role models in many of the mothers I've come to know.

Rules and reasons and right are harder to find. They can be elusive and variable, clear one moment but not the next, even though what has changed may be subtle. Truths do not always transfer from one person to another. Defining my life is not what I thought it would be. It is harder—and yet, when the light comes in just the right way, it is so very simple.

The boys who had been hurt in the gang fight walked to the ambulance themselves. The paramedics wanted to put the big one with the head injury on a stretcher, but he refused. They walked through the lobby in the same confident way they walked through the housing development. A few people looked up as they passed, but not many, and those that did looked right back down again. It didn't take long in the inner city to learn that it was safest to mind your own business. Besides, the arrival of ambulances was common, one of those everyday details of life that goes on in the background.

The fourteen-year-old nodded to me as he left. You're welcome, I nodded back. Not that I did anything, I thought with sadness and shame. I treated an endlessly deep wound with gauze bandage and adhesive tape. I did nothing that would save him.

Two

The nine-month-old baby in Room One had a temperature of 104.5°F. I couldn't find any reason for the fever during his physical examination, like an ear infection or a runny nose, so I'd sent him to the lab for blood tests and urine tests. While we waited for the results, his mother was bathing him in a big blue plastic tub filled with tepid water, trying to bring down the fever. The baby was not pleased with the bath. For a while, he screamed, but then he just sat there with his lower lip out, whimpering, while his mother wet a washcloth and then squeezed the water out of it onto him, again and again. The water made little rivers down his smooth dark skin, across his round belly. As his mother leaned down to talk to him, trying to get him to smile, the ends of her long black hair fell forward into the water in the tub. She didn't notice. All of her attention was on the baby and covering all of his hot skin with water.

The eight-year-old boy in Room Two had asthma and was getting an aerosol treatment. He sat stiffly on the exam table, holding the mouthpiece gingerly between his lips, scowling at his mother who kept telling him to take deeper breaths. She had been impatient to leave from the moment she entered the clinic; she sat in the chair with her coat on and her purse on her lap. The boy's asthma wasn't very bad and he'd probably be able to leave after the aerosol, which was good because we needed to free up a room. The waiting room was full of patients, and many more were expected to show up later that afternoon.

At Martha Eliot the pediatricians and nurse practitioners spend each morning or afternoon session seeing either sick children or well children—the well children being the ones there for physicals and other routine appointments, or what is called "well child care" in pediatrics. This was done for ease of scheduling, and also perhaps to allow the provider to get into one "mode" of seeing patients. The sick visit appointments are called "Triage" appointments. The appointments are brief; about fifteen minutes are allotted, but as there are usually more patients than appointment slots, it ends up being more like five to ten minutes unless a patient needs observation. In that case they sometimes end up staying for hours. Triage appointments are relatively straightforward, organized around a particular symptom or illness. There is no such thing as an entirely straightforward Triage session, of course, because the lives of our patients are not straightforward. Many are living either in poverty or close to its edge, and the stress and paucity of resources make handling life's daily challenges harder. I understand that now, and it doesn't bother me when a visit that should have been easy becomes complicated. At the beginning I didn't understand, and it bothered me.

I went into Room Three, to see a four-year-old girl with a stomachache. At least that's what her mother had said when she made the appointment—she said that the girl had a bad stomachache and had vomited twice. But the girl, who had pigtails and big round cheeks, was happily playing with a doll on the exam table. She didn't have a fever, and didn't wince at all when I pressed on her stomach.

I turned to the mother, an overweight dark-haired woman who was holding an infant. "She seems fine," I said. "When did she last say her stomach hurt?"

The mother looked sheepish. "Well, yesterday morning."

"Yesterday morning?"

"I know, I figured it was a virus or something, but the nurse at the shelter where we been staying said she had to see the doctor. I couldn't get a ride here yesterday, so we came today."

"Do you need a note for the shelter?"

"Yeah, would you mind? They get mad if you don't have a note. I don't want to get kicked out—we got no place else to go right now."

I scribbled a note, and got the girl a sticker. When I started work at Martha Eliot I would have been annoyed that the girl was there, because she was fine and her mother knew it and she was tying up an appointment we could have used for a sicker child. But now I am not annoyed. You can't just bring your kids to the doctor when you live in a shelter, unless it is within walking distance of the doctor's office. Most people in shelters don't have cars, and the kids aren't usually sick enough for ambulances, so either they take public transportation, which isn't the greatest if the kid is sick (especially if they are vomiting), or they try to get a ride, which can be hard to do on short notice. And because there are a lot of people living in close quarters in a shelter, the staff there rightfully want to know what is going on with the child and whether it is contagious. There is no point in being annoyed. A certain number of unnecessary appointments are inevitable in any pediatric practice, as children sometimes get better after the appointment is made. We just have more than average. Being annoyed would be a waste of energy.

I checked the lab tests on the baby with the high fever; the results showed that he most likely had a virus. His fever had come down enough to take him out of the bath; he was dressed and looked much happier on his mother's lap. The mother's wet hair was gathered back in a ponytail now; she was relaxed and smiling. I gave her a prescription for medication to keep the fever down and told her to make an appointment for the next day so we could check on him. She lived nearby and had a phone, so I figured that even if she didn't show up, we could find her.

We never really know if patients are going to show up. Even the ones who are incredibly reliable, the ones who have never missed an appointment before, sometimes don't come. They come, usually, when the children are very sick or hurt, but the follow-up appointments and the physicals are very often missed. It's not that they don't care or don't understand. It's just that life is different around here, and things get in the way of going to the pediatrician, things like transportation, money, or not having someone to watch the other children. Then there are appointments that often take precedence out of necessity, like appointments at Housing or the Welfare office, appointments that are infamous for their long waits. And then there's the simple reality that when life is difficult, people just plain old forget about appointments.

I take this for granted now, and incorporate it into my plans for patients. I make plans that allow for the possibility that I will never see the patient again.

The little boy with asthma sounded much better. He no longer sat stiffly; instead, he leaned back on his elbows and kicked the side of the exam table. His mother asked if they could leave soon—she had two more to pick up from school in twenty minutes, and she needed to cash her welfare check so that she could buy food for dinner. I asked Alison, the nurse, to go in to make a follow-up appointment for him and make sure that he had enough medication. The mother had told me she did, but she was so anxious to go that she might not have been entirely truthful. The mothers are always more truthful with Alison; I don't know whether it is something about the way she asks the questions or just that they trust her more.

Alison started at the clinic just before I did, and is still there. She is in her thirties, thin, and blond. Her clothes and her manner are casual and direct; she speaks perfect Spanish after spending time working in Latin America. The other nurse, Helen, who left in 1996 to hike the Appalachian Trail, had worked in Peru and spoke the musical, incredibly polite Spanish of Peruvian villages. Helen had short dark hair and a wiry, athletic body that was always in motion. The chaos of the clinic is felt most by the nurses, who are constantly barraged by patients and their parents in the hallway and by the constant phone calls. The pediatricians can hide for a moment or two, can choose to take a call later, can exert at least a little control over their time. The nurses have no such options.

I looked through the stack of charts in the plastic box on the door of Room Two, where the nurse puts the charts of the patients she has screened, the patients who are waiting to see me. Two-year-old with cough. Six-year-old with sore knee. Ten-month-old with diarrhea. I looked at the place where the secretary put the charts of patients who had yet to be screened; there were three or four charts there. It was going to be a long afternoon.

Now, I just take my breath and jump in. But at the beginning, when I first came to work at Martha Eliot, I was completely over-whelmed. I was fresh out of pediatric residency training, where the work was very different. I was busy and there were harrowing moments and it was stressful, but there were lots of conferences and rounds where we could sit and rest and discuss medicine. It was orderly, usually, and very supported. I was part of a collective brain, many people thinking together about patients. There was always somebody more senior looking over my shoulder, checking my work, making sure nothing was forgotten, helping me through. There were senior physicians and specialists always available; every patient was discussed at least once a day and often much more than that. My tasks were limited and clear. For example, the oncologists decided on the chemotherapy for the children with cancer, while I took care of their mouth sores and fevers in the way the oncologists told me to. The allergists told me which medications I should use for the asthmatics. The gastroenterologists told me what diets to give the children with intestinal problems, and what tests to order. I did make decisions on my own, but only ones I was comfortable making, and help was never more than seconds away.

When I went to Martha Eliot I left that behind. There were

other pediatricians around to discuss patients with, most of the time, but often they were equally stumped, or too busy to really listen or help. I was expected to make medical decisions alone.

There was nothing wrong with this; after all, I'd finished three years of training in a hospital with an excellent reputation. It was reasonable to expect me to be capable—and for the most part, I was. But I was scared—scared of missing something important, scared of forgetting something, scared of being in a situation where I didn't know what to do. I did not enjoy my independence, at least not at first.

And what made it harder was that there were aspects of practicing medicine at Martha Eliot that residency did not prepare me for.

Residency didn't cover the cultural aspects of practicing medicine, which were especially an issue with the Latin American patients. I spoke Spanish, so I mistakenly thought that I would be fine—but what I didn't fully realize was that culture is much more than just language. Many of the patients had beliefs about health and illness that were entirely different from mine.

In my first week at Martha Eliot I met a mother from the Dominican Republic who was very unhappy with me when I told her that her son didn't need treatment for grinding his teeth. Alison came into the room to get a suture-removal kit out of a drawer as I was saying that this was not something to worry about.

"Don't you think he needs any tests?" the mother asked in Spanish.

Alison tapped me on the shoulder. "Could I talk to you a second?" she said. We went outside the room.

"In the Dominican Republic they think that when people grind their teeth it means that they have parasites," she said. "Most of them don't, or if they do, it's probably just coincidence. But this mother isn't going to leave until you agree to check her son for parasites."

I went back into the room, humbled, and gave the mother the vials and lab forms for stool samples.

It wasn't just the Latin American patients. There were lots of families, of all ethnicities, who looked at health and illness differently from the way I'd been taught to look at them, families whose backgrounds were different from mine in all sorts of ways. Culture is always powerful.

The support staff became my teachers. Marta, one of the nursing assistants, is from Puerto Rico. She has been at Martha Eliot for years, and has strong opinions about how things should be and be done. She is quick to correct my Spanish or tell me when I've done something else wrong, sometimes in front of the family—but she will do absolutely anything to help and is wonderful with the families. She understands the underpinnings of both small and big things in the various Latino cultures we dealt with, she knows many of the families extraordinarily well, and they trust her completely. The other nursing assistant who was there when I started was Sarah, an older, graceful African-American woman who had been at the clinic even longer and retired a couple of years ago. She didn't speak Spanish, but she really didn't need to—she knew how to communicate without words. She could calm any baby, and all the children loved her. And she knew the life stories of so many of the families who came to the clinic; they were her neighbors, her friends, and she had watched them grow up. She had a wonderful ability to get inside people's heads and understand why they did the things they did. Gently, quietly, she would give me hints about people, helping me to know what to do.

Logistical issues seemed endless at Martha Eliot, something I was also unprepared for. There were never enough appointment slots, we were frequently short staffed, there weren't enough exam rooms when things got busy, there was only about two feet square of work space for each of us in the staff room. We ran out of immunizations intermittently, out of diapers and other supplies often. There was constant paperwork: lab forms, requisitions, referral forms, billing forms, doctors' orders forms from visiting nurses.

Betty, the secretary, guided me through this. She taught me the intricacies of scheduling and the user-hateful computer system, as well as which form needed to be done when and where extras were kept. She sits at the desk at the front of Pediatrics, handling phone calls, preparing charts, dealing with the steady flow of people who come to the clinic wanting all sorts of things. She is in her thirties, an attractive African-American woman with a dry sense of humor and a sharp tongue. She handles everything with equanimity, and she makes it clear that she is too busy to deal with any nonsense. She'll tell you what to do, briefly and without expression, and then go back to her work.

Cost had never really been an issue during residency; it was not generally taken into account in designing treatment plans. It's not that all of the patients I encountered in the hospital had insurance, because I'm sure many of them didn't and went home with huge bills. We simply weren't taught to ask. It is a bit different now as insurance companies, especially health maintenance organizations, are requiring that they be consulted in hospital plans, but when I was in training this practice was only just beginning to emerge. We wrote orders for whatever test or medication we wanted the patient to have, guided by what we thought was medically necessary—or medically interesting. Patients existed for us as clinical dilemmas, not necessarily as people with ongoing lives. The fact that we rarely saw patients again after they were discharged reinforced this view.

At Martha Eliot issues of cost and insurance are always taken into account—probably because we see patients again and again and have a clear concept of their ongoing lives. Also, we see the children come back still sick when their parents can't afford the medication we prescribe, for unlike inpatients who get their medications from the hospital pharmacy and are billed for it later, the local pharmacies want money or an insurance card before giving over anything. Never write a prescription, the staff told me, unless you are sure the family has the means to fill it—and frequently they didn't. There were samples of some medications in the med room, from drug companies and from the pharmacy at Children's, which helped. But there weren't samples of everything, and I began to find myself looking for cheaper ways of doing things: cheaper antibiotics, cheaper ointments, home recipes for whatever I could find a home recipe for. Instead of designing the ideal medical treatment, I assessed what was possible and took it from there, making compromises I hadn't been taught about making.

Compromises are a big part of practicing medicine at Martha Eliot. Rarely is something perfect, exactly as it could or should be. That doesn't mean it's not good medicine, because it is good medicine. We take very good care of the people who come to the clinic; I know this clearly now, after working here a few years and seeing all that we can do, all the ways we can help. It's just that problems are more complicated here, and solutions become more complicated too.

I didn't learn what to do in a day, or a week, or a month. I learned over longer than that, in bits and pieces, from the staff and from the patients. I learned on my feet. This kind of learning was very familiar to me. In residency I learned on my feet, thrown into challenging situations where I had to pull together what I knew and what I felt and figure out what to do. Since my daughter was born I'd discovered that parenthood was much the same way. Most of the best things we do in our lives are learned on our feet, because they are too hard to teach and because there are so many different ways to do them.

The two-year-old with a cough had a cold, and was sent out with a sample of cough medicine. The six-year-old with the sore knee had bumped it on the playground, and needed no treatment except rest. The ten-month-old with diarrhea had a virus; we sent him and his mother home with oral rehydration instructions, telling her to call if he was any worse.

The others were more of the same—another child with asthma,

one with an ear infection, a couple with fevers, another with diarrhea, another with a cough. It was a fairly typical afternoon, with
typical childhood illnesses. Not that things are entirely typical at
Martha Eliot. One of the children with a cough needed to be
tested for tuberculosis because one of the people in the over-
crowded apartment he lived in had just been diagnosed with this.
The second child with diarrhea had a sixteen-year-old mother
who had been feeding him cheeseburgers and French fries during
his illness, not understanding that this might not be the best diet
for him. The child with the ear infection had been given a prescription the week before for the same thing, but his father was too
proud to tell us that he couldn't afford it, and the infection had
grown much worse.

The last patient of the afternoon was a four-year-old who came
in with her foster mother, holding the woman's hand tightly as she
was led into the exam room. She was African-American, small, and
skinny. Her jeans were fastened around her waist with a shoelace
as a makeshift belt; they were much too big. She wore a faded print
shirt with a hole in front.

The foster mother apologized for the little girl's clothes.

"DSS brought her to me yesterday," she said. "I haven't had
time to take her shopping. I wanted to bring her here first because
of her fever."

I asked if the Department of Social Services had told her anything
about the child's medical history. The foster mother shook her head.

"All I know is that she was abused," she said under her breath.
"They didn't tell me anything else."

The woman was an experienced foster mother who also had
two children of her own. She came to the clinic often.

"I noticed the fever last night," she said. "It seemed like something was hurting her. I gave her Tylenol but it didn't seem to help
much. I ended up holding her most of the night."

The little girl looked up at me, terrified, as the foster mother put her up on the exam table. Alison had taken her temperature; it was 103°F. Her eyes were huge, and they watched my every move. Her bony hands gripped the edge of the table tightly. I listened to her heart and lungs; they were normal. I asked her to open her mouth. She did and then flinched; when I only shined the light in she seemed surprised.

"Okay, now let's check your ears," I said.

"This may be where the problem is," said the foster mother. "She kept touching her right ear last night."

The girl let me look in her left ear with my otoscope, but when I approached her right ear she started to cry and moved away from me, covering her ear with her hand.

"Let me help," said the foster mother. She climbed up on the table and put the girl on her lap. She wrapped one arm around the girl's torso so she couldn't move her arms, and with the other hand, she held the girl's head against her chest. The girl started to scream. Quickly, I looked in her right ear; it was very infected. I nodded at the foster mother, who let go.

The little girl's screams suddenly turned into sobs. She buried her head in the foster mother's breasts and her small, thin arms wrapped around her. She held this stranger, this woman she had known for only a day, as if she had always known her. She held this stranger tight as if she never wanted to let her go.

I wrote out a prescription for antibiotics and handed it to the foster mother, who put it in her pocket, thanking me. Still holding the little girl, she got up off the table, carrying her out the door.

"It's going to be okay," she said to her softly. "It's going to be okay."

I stood in the doorway, watching them. Alison came up next to me.

"She's a good mother," she said. "That kid is lucky."

Luck, I have learned, is defined differently sometimes.

Three

The boy looked at me angrily. He was seven years old, and he sat on the exam table with his arms crossed in front of him. He had put the hospital gown on after much persuasion, but he would not open his mouth. I was feeling annoyed.

His dirty jeans, high-top sneakers, and the sweatshirt that was much too small for him lay next to him on the table. He wanted them nearby; it was a condition for his remaining on the table. I figured that he wanted them within reach for easy escape. His brown arms and legs were thin but strong, like those of a small animal. Not a young animal—he was more like an old bobcat. His eyes were full of knowing too much.

His sister sat on the chair next to the exam table. She was ten years old and her clothes were dirty too, but her hair was neatly braided and her face was clean. She looked at me apologetically.

"Please open your mouth," she said to her brother. She reached up and touched his leg. He didn't acknowledge her touch, but he seemed to relax, ever so slightly. "The doctor just wants to look."

The little boy hadn't been to a doctor in more than three years. He had no idea what I was going to do to him, I realized, and no longer felt annoyed.

The boy looked at his sister and then slowly opened his mouth. I took the otoscope off the wall, pulled the earpiece off, and shined the light into his mouth. His molars were black instead of white; he had such bad cavities that the teeth were nothing but fragile shells with black holes in the middle. No wonder he didn't want to open his mouth.

I took a deep breath and turned around to look at his mother.

She was sitting in the corner by the big metal desk, looking out the window. There was nothing to see; the window looked out at the back wall of one of the buildings of the housing development. Yet she stared intently. She was a big woman—tall, heavy, with long hands. She wore an old denim coat that smelled like it hadn't been washed in years; an old wool cap with a few small holes in it was pulled down over her ears. Her face was tired and slightly swollen, giving it a blurred appearance. Although she wasn't moving, she seemed slightly unsteady on the chair. She held a newborn baby awkwardly in her lap; he was so tiny and quiet that I kept forgetting that he was there.

They were all there because of him, though. They were there because the hospital found cocaine and heroin in his urine after the EMTs brought him in. He was born at home, on the bathroom floor. The mother never went to the doctor while she was pregnant. The hospital called the Department of Social Services, who told her that if she didn't stop using drugs and start taking care of her children, the children would be taken away from her.

"Miss Johnson," I said. "Joan." She turned back from the window and looked in my direction, if not quite at me. "Does Jamal ever complain about his teeth hurting?"

She looked at the boy for a long time. Then she looked up at me and her eyes were so full of pain that I was startled.

She didn't know, I realized. She couldn't answer my question.

She turned to her daughter, who had been sitting on the edge of her chair, her eyes moving between me and her mother.

"He does," said the girl softly but clearly. "All the time."

My daughter, Michaela, was six months old. I knew everything there was to know about her. I knew every inch of her, every hair, every fold of skin. I knew exactly how she liked her bottle and which toy made her smile the most; I knew which cry meant she was hungry and which cry meant she was tired. I couldn't imagine not knowing that something hurt her all the time. I didn't know how to react to this family, and I certainly didn't know what to say.

So I didn't say anything. I finished examining Jamal, who was sullenly cooperative with prodding from his sister. His clothes were on in a flash when I was done. I filled out cards for Joan to make appointments for him: for the dentist and to get his vision and hearing checked.

"The vision and hearing appointments are routine, and don't need to be right away. But he needs to get to the dentist as soon as possible. If there's any problem getting an appointment soon, let me know and I'll talk to them." I didn't look at her, she didn't look at me. I laid the cards on the desk, and she slid them off into the big front pocket of the denim coat.

The girl's name was Barbara, and it was her turn next. She shooed Jamal out of the room and sat shyly on the exam table in a hospital gown, her eyes following mine, eager to please. She, too, was thin. I wondered how much food was in the house. She had some cavities, but her teeth were nowhere near as bad as her brother's.

"I always brush my teeth," she said to me. "I try to get Jamal to brush his, but he don't like to."

I looked over at Joan. She had gone back to staring out the window. The baby's eyes were open, looking up at nothing in that unfocused newborn baby way. Joan held him loosely; his head flopped back slightly over her arm.

I finished examining Barbara, whose eyes still carefully followed mine.

"Uh," she said.

"Yes?"

"Am I, uh, uh . . ."

"Yes?"

She took a deep breath. "Am I gonna get my period soon?"

I smiled. "Within the next year or so, I think," I said.

She grinned. "Great," she said. "I can't wait."

"Why?" I asked.

Her voice was soft but clear. "Because then I'll have something to talk about," she said.

"I'm sure you have lots of things to talk about," I said. "You don't need to get your period to have something to talk about."

A shadow passed over her face—an expression of doubt, maybe, or sadness—and then it was gone. She blushed and her eager eyes looked away for a few seconds before coming back to follow mine.

The nurse from Jamal Johnson's school called me a few days later to say that she still hadn't received his health form and that if he didn't get it in he was going to be excluded from school.

I clearly remembered handing it to Joan. She had shoved it into the baby's diaper bag. I told her it was important. I wasn't sure she really heard me. I told the nurse I would send another to her in the mail. I asked how Jamal was doing in school.

"Well, you know," she said, "it's not easy when kids come in like he did, after the school year has started. That plus the fact that he should have started last year, so he's in with first graders who are younger and smaller than he is. He's not making much effort so far, but it's early yet."

When I had asked Joan why she didn't enroll Jamal in school until the Department of Social Services told her to, she shrugged.

"I just didn't," she said. "I guess it was the drugs. I was busy with them, and I didn't think about it."

Barbara scowled at Joan, obviously angry at her mother's easy admission of guilt. Joan looked at her and shrugged again.

Barbara had her mother's big eyes and gentle nose. She wore her many shoulder-length braids gathered at the nape of her neck with a frayed purple ribbon. She was always alert, always watchful.

Jamal was always alert, too, but his alertness was different. He watched everything going on in the room around him. He watched the doors and the windows. He walked slowly, shuffling, dragging behind—but he could move very quickly if startled. He looked at his mother frequently, but only when she wasn't looking at him. When she looked at him he'd quickly look away. When she talked to him he often didn't respond, although you could tell by his shoulders and his eyes that he was listening. If he did respond, he was usually rude. Joan did not react to his rudeness. She just looked at him sadly.

Joan and I didn't talk much for a long time after we met. Each time she came in with one of the children, I'd ask questions politely and briefly about how she was doing; she would answer equally politely and briefly. She kept every appointment, did everything she was told to do. I knew, because I was checking. I was angry at her, angry for the children, and she knew it.

I tried to hide it. I tried to be impartial. But I knew that she heard the anger in my voice, saw it in my eyes. I could tell by the way she looked away from me, by the way she avoided speaking to me. It felt like she was trying to melt into the walls when we were in the same room.

I knew that drug addiction was an illness. I knew there was more to stopping than just deciding to stop. I'd learned all that in medical school. But when I looked at the children, knowing wasn't the same as understanding. They were so beautiful and blameless, and yet they hung on the edge of destruction. They deserved more. They deserved a mother who didn't use drugs, who could give them support, attention, food, a clean place to play and sleep. They deserved someone who could really take care of them. I wished that DSS would take them and put them into foster care.

Joan's baby, Timothy, started wheezing when he was four months old. He'd had a bad cold, and Joan brought him to the clinic because she said that he was "breathing funny." When I listened to his chest I heard a little bit of a wheeze, but he was breathing comfortably. I wrote a prescription for Ventolin, a medication we use to treat wheezing; Joan took it from me almost reluctantly, staring at it.

"You need to go right to the pharmacy after you leave here to get that filled," I said sternly.

"I will," said Joan somewhat blankly, carefully putting the prescription into her pocket.

"Here's the phone number to call to talk to one of us if he gets any worse during the night," I said, giving her the photocopied sheet explaining the on-call system. She put it into her pocket, without changing her expression.

"And he needs to come back to the clinic tomorrow morning so that we can check him again," I said, again sternly. I didn't know how to read her blankness, and I was worried that she might not give him the medicine or call.

When she brought Timothy back the next day he was worse. Joan was clearly worried.

"I been giving him the medicine, and it helps for a while, but then he go back to breathing like this."

She cradled the baby in her arms, no longer loosely. His chest rose and fell quickly, and with each breath I could see his ribs as he used all the muscles in his chest to breathe. He had been born small because the cocaine had damaged the placenta; he was gaining weight well now but he was still smaller than most babies his age. His eyes were wide open, staring up at his mother; he looked uncomfortable and frightened.

"Why didn't you call?" I said.

"I don't got a phone," she mumbled. "I knocked on the neighbors' doors, but they weren't home."

I got the oxygen tank, set up a Ventolin aerosol, and gave it to Joan to hold close to his face so that he would breathe it in. She took it from me clumsily, but held it exactly as I showed her. She leaned down as he breathed in the medicine, whispering softly to the baby, tender things I could barely hear over the hissing of the aerosol. She had lost weight; the denim coat, still unwashed, hung more loosely on her. Her skin was sallow, her shoulders slumped.

Usually I leave the room while a child gets an aerosol, to see more patients or do other work. That time I sat there, watching them, watching her hold him and whisper to him, watching him nestle into her. She held him against her body, the fingers of her free hand stroking him softly as she held him. He stared desperately at her face, as if he wanted to climb inside it, back inside her. When she whispered to him he opened his mouth, silently answering her.

There was something that held me there with them. She is his mother, I thought. He doesn't understand what she has done to herself or to him, and he doesn't care. Neither did the others, even though they were angry. What they wanted, more than any of the many things that they deserved, was to be with her, and to have her love.

And I realized, as I sat there, that Joan was doing the very best she could. That wasn't true before and it might not be true tomorrow, but right now it was true.

After another aerosol and a dose of steroids, Timothy was much better. His chest began to rise and fall more slowly, his eyes closed, and he fell asleep peacefully in Joan's arms.

I sat down at the desk and wrote a prescription for more of the steroids.

"How much does that cost?" asked Joan in a small voice.

"Oh, I don't know, about ten dollars," I said. "But it's okay, Medicaid covers it."

"I don't got Medicaid," she said.

"Why not?" I had assumed she did; most of the poor single mothers who came to the clinic had Medicaid for their children. The ones who didn't were the illegal immigrants, or the mothers with jobs, who often had no insurance because their employer didn't offer it or they couldn't afford the family plans.

"I got some money when Barbara and Jamal's father died, like an inheritance, you know? I spent it all but they say I gotta prove I spent it and I can't."

"How much was it?"

She looked down. "A few thousand."

"What did you spend it on?"

She turned away. "I lived on it for a while," she said quietly. "Mostly, I spent it on drugs."

I had remarkably little reaction to this. I wasn't surprised.

"How did you buy the Ventolin?"

"I borrowed money from my mother. That little bottle cost like thirteen dollars."

"Can you borrow from her again?"

"Not ten dollars, no. She don't got nothin' left. She's waiting for her welfare check. We's supposed to be gettin' one too, but it hasn't come. We spent everything on groceries the other day."

"Is there anybody else . . . ?"

Joan shook her head. She looked sad and very tired.

This wasn't good. If the baby continued wheezing he was going to need more medication and possibly a machine to do aerosols at home. He needed medical insurance.

"Maybe your DSS worker could help you sort the Medicaid problem out. What was her name again?"

"It used to be that Diane person. But she said I was going to get a new one, and I haven't heard from anybody in a long time."

"You're kidding," I said.

She shook her head. Her face darkened, and she frowned. "I been clean," she said.

"No, it's not that," I said, a little flustered. "I just think that you might need more help." It was as if she was set up to fail. With no money to feed her children or buy medicines for them, with nobody there to support and encourage her, how would she ever stay off drugs?

I reached into my pocket and got out two five-dollar bills, which I laid on the desk near her. "Here's some money for the steroids," I said. "I'll call DSS and see if there's some way of helping with the Medicaid."

She looked at the crumpled bills uncertainly.

"Go ahead, take it," I said. "He needs the medicine." I wasn't being generous, I was being practical.

"Thanks," she mumbled, and put the bills in her pocket.

"I'd like to see him back tomorrow," I said. She nodded and began to dress the baby.

I stood up to leave the room, then stopped.

"How did Jamal and Barbara's father die?" I asked.

"He got shot," she said without looking up from the snaps on the baby's clothes.

Four

During that first summer at Martha Eliot, I found myself frequently losing track when I was doing well child care. I lost track of what I was supposed to do next all the time. During residency, I had spent one afternoon a week doing well child care, but I never had to see more than four patients in the afternoon. At Martha Eliot I was expected to see ten to fourteen patients in a three-hour session. I had to talk to them and their families, examine them, figure out what lab tests or services they needed, give shots, do paperwork, and write in charts. Then there were the endless phone calls, lab results to check, and correspondence with consultants. The support staff, the nurses and nursing assistants, helped out a lot. They weighed and measured, asked some screening questions, stamped up lab forms, minded stray children, and did health education with the parents, but still, the workload was tremendous, much more than I expected. And there was no easing into it; from the start, I was fully booked. I found myself running from patient to patient, from task to task, relying on the staff to point me in the right direction. I felt like I was in a pinball machine.

"How can I be fully booked?" I asked Betty. "I only just started. I'm not anybody's doctor—I don't have any patients."

Betty raised her eyebrows and said dryly, "You've been fully booked for a month. Doesn't matter if you're anybody's doctor. You're the only one who had appointments. Soon as I put you in the computer, those appointments were filled. In fact, I think you're overbooked."

During residency, I felt as if who I was didn't matter. I was sim-

ply a body, someone to call to put in the IV or order the medications or take care of the crisis, interchangeably filling the never-
ending needs of the hospital. I was "the intern," then "the junior,"
then "the senior." I was not particularly Dr. McCarthy. I accepted
this as an inevitable part of residency; how could any of the hospital staff invest in really getting to know me when I was only on
their ward for a month at a time, and in three years I would be
gone entirely?

But I thought that once I left residency it would change. Once I
left it would matter who I was; I would be Dr. McCarthy and not
interchangeable. What I didn't anticipate was that the never-ending
needs of the clinic were just as great as those of the hospital, and the
turnover in physicians was such that patients didn't expect me to
stay. Once again I was interchangeable: good as any other, not
worth getting to know.

It's different now. I will always be interchangeable to some, but
for most now I am not. It took a long time, though, and more
effort than I would ever have predicted.

I'd lose track of the Spanish all the time. My Spanish was actually pretty good; I'd studied it in high school, and during medical
school and residency I had developed a wide medical vocabulary. I
encountered enough Spanish-speaking patients during my training so that I practiced the language frequently, and I became con-
versant. But at Martha Eliot I was out of my league.

My medical vocabulary was fine when children were brought in
for illnesses or injuries, but well child care was entirely another
matter. Families wanted to talk about other things besides fever or
vomiting or diarrhea. They wanted to talk about toilet training
and behavior problems and school, about all sorts of things that
required words I'd never learned. And Spanish isn't just one language, of course. Mothers from the Dominican Republic and
mothers from Guatemala use different words for breast-feeding
and for naughtiness; they have different ways of phrasing questions

and talking to their children. The Latino families who come to Martha Eliot are mostly from the Dominican Republic, but we have families from most Central American and South American countries as well. So many times I'd look at them blankly, or they'd look at me blankly, and we'd try to find a different word, a different way, in Spanish or English, to understand one another. Sometimes we could, but sometimes we couldn't.

I would sit and listen to all the words that people were saying to me, and try to piece them together so that I could understand them. Usually I could understand most of what they were saying, but sometimes I'd only catch a few words. Then I'd have to try to figure out what was going on by the context, or the gestures and facial expressions.

It wasn't just the Spanish that made me lose track, though. I'd lose track when I was speaking English, too. I'd lose track of what people were telling me, because there were so many problems, so many things to think about. Situations changed frequently. Families always seemed to be moving; the addresses and phone numbers never lasted long. The composition of families changed, as children were shuffled among relatives, or in and out of foster care, as fathers came and went and teenagers left home. At times people could afford food and medicine, at times they couldn't. I had to know these things, to know what was feasible and what was needed, and to know what was being mirrored in the children.

In pediatrics there is a lot of emphasis on what we call "social history": where and how people live, what they believe in, what supports and resources they have. These are incredibly important in the health of children, because they dictate how the children will be cared for—and they dictate, to a large extent, what sort of people the children will grow up to be. Pediatricians are taught to be nosy, to ask a lot of questions.

The problem was that sometimes after I asked all my questions, I didn't know what to do with the answers.

*   *   *

A sixteen-year-old mother of a newborn burst into tears and told me that her mother was kicking her out of the house because she was angry with her for getting pregnant, that the baby's father was in jail, and she had nowhere to go. And why, she wanted to know, did the baby cry all the time? She was so, so tired that all she did was cry too.

A four-year-old with asthma had been sick several times over the preceding few weeks, more than he had ever been in the past. When his father brought him in for a physical I asked if anything was different at home that might be causing the increase in his wheezing. The father told me that the family had been evicted from their apartment and had moved in with his wife's brother. There were eight of them living in a two-bedroom apartment which was poorly heated, and his wife's brother had a cat. All of this could make the boy's asthma worse. There was nothing he could do about it, the father told me. They had no choice.

A mother of a two-year-old and an infant, a quiet woman in her early twenties, was quieter than usual and asking me for the children's medical records, "in case I have to leave town." When I asked her what was going on she said there was nothing, but finally she told me that her husband had been beating her and was threatening her life.

I had asked for the information; supposedly, I had wanted to know. And now the information was there, lying in front of me, and had to be dealt with.

I quickly learned what options I had. The Human Services department of the clinic had people to help families, either with advocacy or psychological help or both. There were outreach programs. There were visiting nurses, who were usually happy to work with me to find a medical excuse, like checking on a newborn's weight gain, to visit a family. There were churches and other community resources; there were hotlines and lawyers and, when necessary, there was the police.

I also quickly learned, however, that my options had limitations. The caseworkers, social workers, and psychologists in Human Services had huge caseloads, and could help only so much. The outreach programs were stretched to their limits. The visiting nurse could visit only so many times before the insurance wouldn't pay. And so it went. People wanted to help, but they were busy and under all sorts of constraints. And the families had to want to be helped, which sometimes they didn't, either because they wanted their privacy, or because they were proud, or because changing their lives took a will they couldn't muster.

So I couldn't simply run looking for help, or promise that things would change or even get better. I had to find a response that was real from within myself, a response that would be accepted and possibly helpful.

Finding the response wasn't hard. My response was that I cared, and I wanted to help in whatever way I could. This was what I tried my best to convey. I said it again and again. I asked lots of questions and listened intently, trying with everything I did to convey my interest and concern. I reached out, touched their arms, hugged them when they were upset. I asked them what they thought might help, and offered suggestions, promising them that I would do anything and everything possible.

Having the response be accepted, though, was harder than I expected. It seemed obvious to me that my concern and commitment were genuine; if they weren't, why would I be working at the clinic? But it wasn't that simple. There was an awkwardness, a distance between me and the families that was frustratingly unbreachable.

What do you know, I could see their eyes saying. What do you know of my life? You white-skinned doctor, what could you possibly know? You get in your car at the end of the day and drive away from all of the things we can't get away from. You go home to a life that we will probably never have.

I couldn't argue with the things I saw their eyes saying. The differences were there. I wanted to wipe them away, but I couldn't. And these differences that I wanted to wipe away were parts of me that I would never have dreamed would be a problem. My upper-middle-class background had always opened doors for me, but at Martha Eliot it was closing doors between me and families. I had always been proud of my Ivy League education, but now it made me someone out of touch and reach—if it meant anything to them at all. Many of the Latino families had never heard of Princeton or Harvard.

Who would I be without these things? I found myself wondering. Quite possibly I wouldn't be at the clinic, for without them I might not have been a doctor, or I might have been so overloaded with loans that I couldn't afford to work at an inner-city clinic. It seemed like a catch-22, an impossible situation. But maybe, I thought, not all of the differences are intrinsic or important. Maybe there are some that I can put aside, or at least hide.

I found myself dressing down—not so casually that it appeared I didn't take my job seriously, but I didn't wear anything expensive or flashy. I wore my wedding ring and inexpensive earrings, but no other jewelry. I didn't talk about my background; I didn't talk about myself at all. I didn't have an office, so hanging diplomas wasn't an issue, but I probably wouldn't have hung them if I could.

I watched the mannerisms and gestures of the families, trying to copy them. I listened carefully to the language, both Spanish and English, learning the slang the families used, so I could talk like they did. I wanted to blend in.

Within a few months, I was losing track less. I had learned my way around and the pace became natural; I got into patterns that allowed me to move quickly and comfortably through a busy session. My Spanish got better. I developed a whole set of "speeches" in Spanish on well child care topics like safety and toilet training and time-outs that I could use, and I gathered enough vocabulary that I could discuss just about any topic. I didn't understand every single word the Latino families said to me, but I understood much more.

I lost track of the issues less. I became more familiar with them, and so less intimidated. As I got to know the families, I became able to anticipate what they might say to me, and so I was less often caught off guard. And as I got to know the available resources better, I felt less helpless. Only a little less—I still feel helpless—but less enough.

The only part that didn't become easier was blending in. Trying to look and talk like the patients didn't do the trick—not that I was doing it particularly well. The fact was that I didn't look or talk like them. The fact was that I was different, whether I liked it or not. As they got to know me, the families were more pleasant and friendly, but the distance was still there.

What really frustrated me was that as I got to know people better, I didn't feel that different from them. As I got to know them better, it seemed that we wanted the same things from our lives: to make a comfortable existence, to raise our children and find our way in the world, to be loved. Our stories get played out in different ways, depending on the context, but they are so very much the same story.

Differences can be like thorn-covered branches, keeping the stories apart, keeping them parallel when they might otherwise touch.

Five

y favorite time of the day is the early morning, the very early morning, as the light seeps into the sky. I love the way the morning light touches, softly bringing everything out of the darkness. I love how everything is so quiet, and so very possible.

For the first year of her life Michaela usually woke up at around five in the morning, so often I'd meet the dawn with her in my arms, watching the light bring her out of the darkness as she sucked on her bottle. It would light her dark hair and her full cheeks, and bit by bit reveal her tiny nose, her pink lips, and her long eyelashes, taking my breath away each time. I would sit there, overwhelmed into motionless by her beauty and by my dreams for her. Too soon the light would fill the room, bringing with it the noises, and the work, of the day. The magic moment was gone, at least until the next dawn.

Michaela was born on Valentine's Day of 1991, all ten pounds, five ounces of her bursting into our lives and taking it over completely. Somehow, I had thought of a child as something that you worked into your life. I waddled around the hospital during my pregnancy very much myself except for my big belly and my nausea, planning on being the same after the baby's birth except for a few logistical changes. But then she was born and I was working my life around hers and nothing, nothing would ever be the same.

I was a senior resident at Children's Hospital when she was born. My husband, Mark, was a respiratory therapist there. We met in the neonatal intensive care unit on a fourth of July, beginning a whirlwind romance that led to our marriage about a year later. There was something about his gentleness, his thoughtfulness, his clear goodness that said to me: marry this one. So I did. It was the best decision I have ever made.

Because of the constraints of residency scheduling, I had to go back to work when Michaela was only seven weeks old. Uneasy about leaving her with a baby-sitter or in day care, we patchworked together a crazy schedule. I was working sixty or so hours a week, but many of them were nights, and Mark worked shifts which could be moved around, and his mother was willing to help out when despite our best efforts our work hours overlapped . . . it meant elaborate scheduling, frequent "baby pass-offs" in front of the hospital, and essentially never seeing each other. By the time my remaining three months of residency were over we were exhausted and miserable, and fighting all the time. Clearly, our life needed to change if our marriage and our mental health were to remain intact.

I had an offer to work in a private practice as well as at Martha Eliot, but we decided that I should turn it down and only work at the clinic, three days a week. I had signed a contract to write a book about my experiences in medical school and residency, so we figured that not only would I be able to be home more with Michaela, but I could use the time at home to write. Mark continued to work full-time, but went to all twelve-hour shifts instead of eight-hour shifts, and began to work every other weekend. This meant that he only had to work two days during the week and could be home with Michaela when I was working. We still didn't see each other as much as we would have liked, but with my cutback in hours we saw each other much more. Life felt more orderly and normal, and we were able to begin to relax and enjoy each other and Michaela.

On the days he worked Mark left at around six in the morning and didn't get home until after eight in the evening, so my days at home with Michaela were very much alone with her. After her early morning bottle, she usually went back to sleep, giving me some time to have coffee and get dressed and write for a while. Within an hour or so, she would be awake, crying for me from her crib. Then it was time for her baby-food breakfast, and changing, dressing, and organizing for the day. These simple tasks could take me two hours sometimes. She'd play and be slow with eating, I'd have to clean her and the chair and the surrounding floor afterward, then I'd have to hunt for clean clothes in the unfolded laundry, fight with her to get her clothes on, find her jacket and shoes, pack the diaper bag, check to see if her diaper needed rechanging, and so on.

I had newfound respect, awe even, for the mothers I saw at the clinic who managed two or more children at once with ease, and arrived for their appointments on time. Although I had always considered myself an organized and efficient person, getting myself and one child out of the house to walk to the park was often difficult; the tasks of taking care of a child were new and awkward to me. I was like a kid learning to ride a two-wheeler, stumbling and off-balance.

I liked taking Michaela to the park whenever the weather was good. It got us out of the confines of the house, which I found I needed. I wasn't exactly claustrophobic, but it was hard to spend day after day in just four rooms, which was all our house had, with nobody to talk to but an infant. Michaela enjoyed the stroller ride, anyway, and I enjoyed the exercise. Long-distance running had been added to the list of previous activities relegated indefinitely to the back burner; opportunities for exercise were few.

We lived in Melrose, a suburb northeast of Boston, where Mark had grown up and where his family still lived. I had always imagined that I would live in the city; I liked the activity, the mix of faces and cultures, and all the things there were to see and do. But instead, I had ended up in suburbia. There were various little reasons, like that the house Mark rented from his stepfather, although small, was bigger and cheaper than my cramped city apartment, parking was easier, there was a tree from which to hang a baby swing, and Mark's big dog would never have adapted to city life. But the biggest reason was Mark's family: his mother, his stepfather, his two brothers and their wives, and the extended family, most of whom lived in or near Melrose.

They were a very close family, which was a new experience for me. My family was scattered around the country, coming together infrequently and awkwardly. It took a while to get used to seeing Mark's family almost every day, sometimes in unexpected visits, sharing meals often, and having facts about our lives that I previously would have considered private become common knowledge. But with Michaela's birth, it all became easier to accept. Mark's mother would show up with dinner for us and diapers for the baby. Mark's sister-in-law, who had a baby a few months older than Michaela, would baby-sit so I could do rounds at the hospital or run some errands. Mark's stepfather would stop by when I needed help with something in the house while Mark was at work, or when there were crises, like the time the bees came in through the air conditioner. And most of all, Michaela's world was filled with people who loved her and would do anything, anything at all for her.

Melrose is an old town, very hilly and rocky, filled with Victorian houses and well-kept yards. It has a Main Street, a city hall, a library, and its own weekly newspaper filled with stories about the school committee, the soccer league, the fund-raising for the senior center. The police reports published in the paper are remarkably tame; there is an occasional attack or theft, but mostly they consist of calls for "suspicious persons" that weren't there when the police arrived, minor vandalism, or music that was being played too loud. There is a country club area with expensive houses, but for the most part it is a middle- and working-class

town, which I liked. I didn't want to raise Michaela amid affluence; I didn't want her to take things for granted.

Not that we could afford to raise her amid affluence. By choosing to do inner-city primary care, and by working part-time, I lowered my salary significantly from what it could have been had I
gone into private practice. And although Mark made a respectable
salary, student loan payments took a big part of his paycheck. We
weren't poor; one week working at Martha Eliot was enough to
make me very grateful for what we had. But we couldn't afford
vacations or anything extra, and buying a house was not going to
happen anytime soon.

The park was a twenty-minute walk away, along residential
streets, up a big hill. We always went to the playground, an
enclosed area set apart from the playing field and basketball court.
The playground was mostly shaded, which was nice in the summer. It had a couple of swing sets and jungle gyms and a large
wood contraption that had slides on either end, various platforms,
and a hanging bridge.

Michaela was too young for most of it, and would be until she
learned to walk, but she liked the baby swings. She could swing for
an hour if I had the patience, which I usually didn't, laughing and
squinting into the sun. I envied her ability to get so completely,
joyfully lost in the simple act of swinging back and forth.

There were always other mothers there with their children, and
we would chat as we pushed our children on the swings or
watched them play. We would talk about things like the price of
diapers, the best sales on children's clothing, the weather, and how
the city should fix up the park. We would share stories about our
children, about our frustrations and the moments that made us
laugh. I liked the chats. They were a nice break from talking to an
infant, and a nice break from talking about medicine.

I rarely told any of the mothers that I was a pediatrician. People
seemed to expect more of me as a parent when they found out that

I was a pediatrician. They expected me to know everything and be perfect at parenting. I did know some things, like the immunization schedule, how to diagnose and treat common infections, and what to do if one of the children fell off a swing. But the problem is, immunizations aren't that frequent, kids don't get sick all that often, and thankfully they rarely fall off swings.

Mark expected me to know everything, too. He was constantly asking me questions: which diaper ointment should he use, how should he mix the rice cereal, what he should do when she cried. Very often, I didn't have the answers. And when I did have them, I was frequently drawing on common sense or baby-sitting experience rather than anything I'd learned in my pediatric training.

There is a whole realm of taking care of children that medical school and residency simply don't teach you. They teach you the scientific stuff: illnesses, the biologic aspects of growth and development, the textbook aspects of behavior, et cetera. But they don't teach you about the hows of feeding and changing diapers, the traumas of colic and teething, what to put in a diaper bag, and all the other small things that fill your day when you take care of a child.

I found myself watching the mothers at the clinic very carefully. Mostly, I would watch their hands. I would watch the way they held and fed their children, the way they dressed them, the way they put on their boots and fastened them into strollers, the way they comforted them. Sometimes the mothers would catch me looking at their hands and they would look down at them and then at me, not understanding. They had no idea how quickly and expertly their hands moved, how easily and effectively they did what needed to be done.

Being a pediatrician had not made being a parent easier. And being a parent had not made being a pediatrician easier, either. I figured that at some point it would, once I could talk from experience about more things than breast-feeding (which I only did briefly because of going back to residency so soon), colic, and changing diapers. But for now, being a parent made being a pediatrician harder.

This hit me immediately when I went back to work as a resident after maternity leave. Suddenly I saw Michaela in every child, and myself in every parent. In a tertiary-care hospital, where so many children have serious illnesses or injuries and a significant portion of my work involved sticking needles into children and otherwise hurting them, my inability to separate made my work incredibly painful. A child with cancer, a frightened mother in the waiting room of the intensive care unit, the screams of a baby whose blood I was drawing . . . these always reduced me to tears.

My feelings certainly cemented my decision to do primary-care pediatrics when I was finished with residency. I needed to get away from the hospital, to somewhere where children were mostly well, or I would cry myself to sleep every night.

They don't teach you in medical school how difficult and scary it can be to be a parent, how small things like a fever or fussiness can feel very important and complex, how it can be overwhelming to be alone with and completely responsible for another human being. I was having difficulty adjusting to this. I would tell myself: it's just a little fever, she looks well, or, it's only colic, there is nothing wrong with her. But I was not easily comforted. The stakes were too high.

Being a pediatrician felt completely different, not only because it was hard to separate but because I understood the import of each bit of advice I gave, each diagnosis I made, each interaction I had with a parent. I understood the tremendous responsibility of my job.

When one or both of us got tired of the park we'd head home, down the big hill, past my mother-in-law's house, up and over curbs. Michaela would often fuss about half of the way back. I would sing to her and pop wheelies with the stroller to keep her amused, but if that didn't work I ended up carrying her on my hip and pushing the stroller one-handed the rest of the way.

Once we were home it was time for lunch and bottle, and then I would rock her to sleep in the rocking chair that took up most of her bedroom. I knew four lullabies, and I would sing them over and over again, putting her into her crib as she began to fall asleep. If she started to cry when I put her in the crib, I'd lean over the railing and sing some more until she fell asleep. Sometimes it would take a long time to get her down for her nap, but I didn't notice and it didn't really matter. Time had a different feel and meaning now.

When she was asleep there was housework to do: picking up toys, doing laundry, cleaning the kitchen, starting dinner. I moved quickly so as to get as much done as possible before my baby awoke and needed me again. I would watch my hands folding undershirt after undershirt, matching socks, cutting vegetables, wiping counters, and I would feel as if somehow they were detached from me, operating independently, because I didn't quite recognize them, or myself. My life was so different since Michaela's birth that sometimes I felt like I was lagging behind it.

When Mark got home at night he would ask me what we had done that day. I would stop, and think, and answer, "We went to the park." It sounded like nothing, and yet my day had been full, and I was exhausted.

The thing is, the tasks and all the small things that filled my days with Michaela were not mindless, although before she was born I would have described them that way. They all mattered: how I responded to her, how I fed her, how I played with her, what kind of home I made for her. It wasn't just baby-sitting or keeping house. It was the making of a person, and this was a very challenging and exhausting job.

Six

I t took me almost a week to finally speak to someone at the Department of Social Services about Joan's Medicaid situation. I called twice for Diane; she didn't call back. I asked the person who answered the phone if they knew how I could find out who Joan Johnson's new worker was; she suggested I speak with Diane's supervisor. I called the supervisor; she didn't call back. I called again; this time, she was in.

"No, Diane Jeffries isn't the worker anymore," said the supervisor. "Ms. Jeffries was just the worker for the investigation."

"So who is the worker now?"

"I don't think it has been assigned yet."

"It hasn't been assigned? The baby is four months old. The 51A was filed when he was born. Why has it taken so long, especially with such a high-risk case?"

There was a long, politic silence before she said, "The case only recently came out of the assessment phase. The person assigned to be the ongoing worker has left, and we are reassigning her cases. Is there a problem with the baby or with Ms. Johnson?"

"No. I mean, yes. I mean, Ms. Johnson is staying clean and taking care of the kids as far as I can tell, but the baby is sick and needs to get on Medicaid."

"She should go to the Welfare office."

"She did. There is a problem with the application, and she needs help."

"Dr. McCarthy, we don't deal with these issues."

"What exactly do you deal with?"

"We deal with child abuse and child welfare."

"Doesn't Ms. Johnson's ability to purchase medicines for her child and otherwise obtain medical care for him have something to do with his welfare?"

There was another long and politic silence.

"I'm sorry, Dr. McCarthy. Perhaps a social worker at your clinic could help her. I will have the new worker get in touch with you."

I was so angry, and so nonplussed, that I couldn't respond. I thanked her, and hung up. I called the Human Services department of the clinic, and was told that if I filled out a referral form, they would discuss it at their weekly meeting and assign someone to see if they could help.

As I dug through the file cabinet for the appropriate form, I wondered what it meant about us as a society that we had turned helping into a dispassionate bureaucracy.

Joan had been coming to the clinic all her life; everyone seemed to know her, and know things about her.

Sarah knew Joan's mother. "They lived on my street," she said. Sarah lived on a tree-lined street in Dorchester of tightly packed Victorian houses in various states of repair.

"Joan's father was a janitor," she said. "Her mother worked as a cashier at the grocery during the day, and at night she cleaned offices. She was a busy woman—we didn't see her much, except on the street and out on the porch some summer evenings. She's really nice, at least she was back then. Joan and her sister Angie were sweet, but their brother Jimmy was trouble. Things started getting real tough for them after Joan's father died."

"How'd he die?" I asked.

"Drank himself to death, I think. That's what the woman who lived next door to them said, although Mrs. Johnson, she just said he'd been ill. The house started falling apart after that—my husband offered to help fix things some, but Mrs. Johnson, she was real proud, she said she could take care of things by herself. But when Jimmy died I think she just gave up."

"What happened to him?"

"Oh, he'd been into drugs for some time. He used to hang with those people with the nice cars and the guns. Those cars were always racing up and down our street, and sometimes we'd hear gunshots. Everybody knew Jimmy was involved, but Mrs. Johnson, she always said that Jimmy was a good boy, that he was just friends with those people and nothing else. But then they found him dead in the Dumpster up the street, shot through the head. He was eighteen."

"Was Joan into drugs then?" I asked.

"No, I don't think so. She was a good student, and worked after school at the Burger King to help out her mother with the money. Her sister Angie, she got pregnant when she was fifteen. She was a scatterbrained girl, not much for taking care of babies, and I know Mrs. Johnson and Joan had to help her out a lot. After Jimmy died, I think it all got to be too much for Mrs. Johnson. She sold the house, moved into an apartment with the girls. Ended up on welfare."

"They live over near Jackson Square," said Betty. "You know the brown triple-decker on that street that goes off Centre Street near the station? They live there. I think they're on the top floor."

"Angie had another baby after they moved into the apartment," said Sarah. "She may be pregnant again for all I know—seems like every time I see her she's on the arm of another guy. She was always way too pretty for her own good, and not very smart. I hear that she runs off a lot with her men friends. I know that she leaves her kids with Mrs. Johnson a lot, 'cause I see her on the street with them."

"Did Joan finish school?"

Sarah shook her head. "She dropped out before they sold the house, to work full-time to help with the bills so that they could keep the house—but it wasn't enough. She kept saying that she was going to go back once they were in the apartment, but, well, what with Angie's babies, and her father's debts, they still had a lot of bills. Mrs. Johnson started to have heart problems so she couldn't work much, and anyway, someone needed to mind Angie's babies. So Joan kept working. She kept working even after she had her babies—Mrs. Johnson would mind them all."

"So when did Joan start using drugs?" I asked.

Betty shrugged. "I think it was sometime after Barbara and Jamal's father got killed. She took that hard. He really doted on her and the kids—you'd see them around Centre Street together, a nice family. He didn't live with them, but he spent a lot of time with them. After he died, we found out that he was a dealer, but I don't know if even Joan knew about that. He kept it real separate from her and the kids. He and his brother had a garage, so she could have thought he got his money from there."

"Who killed him?"

"Other drug dealers, they say," said Betty. "Shot him right in the face."

The next time I took the subway to the clinic, I looked for the brown triple-decker. I walked along Centre Street, a busy street which runs along the housing development after the very modern Jackson Square Station, and then is lined with little shops, many of them with Latino names and merchandise. I saw the street Betty had talked about going off across from the housing development. Two houses in on the left was a triple-decker with old brown shingles, some of them missing. Each floor had a narrow sagging porch in front. A couple of the windows were cracked, and the small backyard was overgrown.

There is a rivalry between the gang at Bromley-Heath and the one at Academy Homes, the housing development that is just across Columbus Avenue from the station. The rivalry gets bloody sometimes. It's never entirely safe around there; a few years ago there was a drive-by shooting outside the station in the afternoon, just as the children were getting out of school. The intended target was hit; the schoolchildren, luckily, were unharmed. It is nearly forgotten now. There are too many shootings to remember them all.

The area around Jackson Square Station is a no-man's-land in the gang war, unprotected and unpredictable. This is where Joan lived; this is where her children were growing up.

Lots of children were growing up there. I'd see them out on their way to school in the morning. Some were with adults, but many were on their own, wearing backpacks, carrying lunch boxes. They walked unhurriedly, like any other children in any other place would. The adults are the same: the mothers with their babies in strollers, the men and women on their way to work, the old ladies walking slowly to the convenience store, the teenagers on the corner. The street was full of people, like any other city street.

It's not that the people out on the street don't know or don't care about the violence. It's just, I think, that life has to go on. So people go out, with a wary eye, with some denial and some hope. Whenever I walk there I am on edge. Living there must mean getting used to feeling on edge, until it becomes normal.

We got Timothy through that first episode of wheezing without having to hospitalize him, but the next time, we weren't so lucky. He started wheezing again about two months later, when he caught another cold. I started him on Ventolin, but the next morning Joan was there the moment the clinic opened, holding the baby in her arms.

"Please, you have to do something," she said.

He was breathing very fast and was very uncomfortable. We tried an aerosol and some steroids but he didn't get appreciably better, so we called an ambulance to take him to Children's Hospital to be admitted.

I went to visit him early the next day, before going to the clinic.

He looked better. Joan was there, lying on a cot next to the crib. It didn't look like she had slept much. She was wearing a faded blue T-shirt and old dirty blue jeans. She sat up as I came in, rubbing her eyes. As she took her hands away, I noticed that she had lovely, high cheekbones. I wondered why I hadn't noticed them before.

She looked at me staring at her, and looked down at herself.

"I know I look awful and that my clothes are dirty," she said. "I've been afraid to take the baby out since he started getting his cold, so I haven't gone to the Laundromat. I been washing the kids' stuff out in the sink, but I just let mine get dirty."

"That's okay," I said.

There was an awkward silence.

I took out my stethoscope, lowered the side of the crib, and listened to Timothy's chest as he slept. Joan stood up next to me, stroking Timothy's cheek.

"He sounds much better," I said. "I'd like him to stay another day, though, unless that's a big problem for you."

"No, it's not a problem," she said. "I'd rather have him here. I'm kind of scared to take him home, after seeing him so bad yesterday."

"I'm going to start him on some regular medication, to see if we can keep him from getting so bad. Does asthma run in your family?"

"Sure does. I had it when I was a kid, and my brother had it too. Does Timothy have asthma?"

"I think so," I said. "It could just be that he got two really bad colds, but it's more likely that it's asthma."

"Shit," she said. She looked up at me. "Cigarette smoke is bad for asthma, isn't it?"

"Yes, it is," I said. "Do you smoke?"

"Sometimes," she said. "But I'll stop, don't worry. I just don't know what I can do about my mother and my sister and my sister's boyfriends."

"Can you get your own apartment?" I asked.

She looked at me like I was crazy. "How?" she asked. "I don't have the money. And I can't get a job now without putting Timothy in day care—my mother can't manage a baby, especially a sick one. There's no way I could get a job that would pay enough for day care and rent and everything else."

"I thought the DSS worker said he was going to help you with housing."

The new DSS worker had finally called; he was a nice guy named Tom Henry, who shared my views on the definition of child welfare. He said that he would see if he could fix the Medicaid problem, and that he would help Joan sign up for public housing.

"I'm on some waiting list," said Joan sourly. "Lady at housing said it could be a couple of years 'fore I get a place."

"Oh," I said. "I didn't realize the waiting list was that long."

"Well, it is," she said. She stopped stroking Timothy's cheek. "You done checking him?" she asked abruptly.

I nodded, and stepped back as she pulled the side of the crib back up.

"I need to get home and make sure the other two get off to school okay," she said. "My mother, she ain't well, and my sister, she ain't always around."

As she reached for the denim coat, which was draped over a chair, I noticed that her hands were shaking.

"Are you okay?" I asked, pointing at her hands.

She looked down at them. "My hands shake when I get tired," she said. "I ain't using, if that's what you're thinking."

"I didn't say that," I said, feeling uncomfortable and defensive. I took a deep breath. I had never actually talked with her about her drug use. I thought I should try.

"How are you doing with that?" I asked awkwardly. "I mean, I know that staying clean isn't easy, and I'm just wondering if you need any help."

"You mean them meetings, the AA and Narcotics Anonymous ones? I go. DSS says I have to. They don't help much, though. I'm doing it by myself." She shifted her weight from one foot to the other. "Can I go now? I really need to get home."

"Sure, of course," I said, and she walked past me out the door.

I didn't know about her life, and I didn't know how to talk to her.

Seven

She moved as if she were dancing, in tiny steps and twirls around the room. Her long legs slid deftly around her brother and sister, who were playing on the exam room floor. Her long black ponytail swung behind her as her delicate arms reached down to pick up the doll her little sister had dropped. The doll was a birthday present that Marta, the nursing assistant, had dug out from a box of donations.

The dancer's name was Daisy, and she was eight years old. The birthday girl, Sharina, was two; she was disturbingly thin, with eyes like saucers and short, dark curly hair. When Daisy gave her the doll she smiled and brought it to Señora Gonzalez, who was holding the baby. Her name was Eliana; she was six months old and so tiny that I could barely see her in the folds of Señora Gonzalez's big shirt.

"*Sí, que muñeca bonita,*" Señora Gonzalez said to Sharina. ("Yes, what a pretty doll.") Her hand caressed the baby's head.

The little boy on the floor, Carlos, was six. He was coloring with some crayons and scrap paper I'd found. He held up a drawing, telling me in Spanish that it was a dinosaur.

They looked peaceful and comfortable, like a happy family—but they weren't. The children's last name was Molina, and they had been with Señora Gonzalez for six days. They were taken from their mother after Eliana was beaten so badly by her mother that she was covered with bruises and had bleeding on her brain. When the police came, called by the neighbors because the children were screaming much more that night than they usually did, there was no food in the filthy apartment. The mother wouldn't say why she beat the baby. The police asked Daisy and Carlos. Daisy wouldn't say anything. Carlos said it was because the baby wouldn't stop crying. The police arrested the mother. She couldn't make bail; she was still in jail.

The mother had a long history of drug abuse, and the family had been monitored by the Department of Social Services since Sharina was born prematurely and tested positive for cocaine. The DSS worker told the police that things had seemed to be getting better; the mother had promised to go to a drug treatment program, and at the last home visit the apartment was clean and there was food in the refrigerator. The worker did admit, though, that it had been almost three months since she'd last seen the family. She had tried, several times, but they didn't have a phone and nobody answered the door when she knocked.

The children were taken to the emergency room at Children's Hospital in an ambulance. Eliana was admitted to the hospital for observation; luckily, the bleeding in her head stopped, and the neurosurgeons said that she would be okay. The other children were found to be malnourished but uninjured, and the social worker brought them from the emergency room to the Gonzalez house. Señora Gonzalez had about two hours' notice. Eliana joined them four days later.

Once Señora Gonzalez had them all, she brought them to the clinic to have them checked. She was an experienced mother and foster mother; she had three grown children of her own and had been taking care of foster children for more than five years, Marta told me. She took it very seriously, Marta said. She made sure that they had their physicals and their dentist appointments, and whatever other appointments she was told they should have. She registered the ones that were old enough for school immediately, so they would miss as few days as possible. She made sure they were clean and well dressed, even if it meant spending her own money on their clothes.

The children were very clean that day, and their clothes were clearly new. The girls, including the baby, were in starched cotton dresses, trimmed with inexpensive lace. Carlos wore corduroys that still had their new pants crease, and a blue cotton sweater.

I asked what medical information she had been given about the children. She raised her eyebrows, dug into her big black purse, and pulled out four "Medical Passports." The big blue cards were supposed to contain information like immunization records, medical problems, allergies, and names of previous doctors. She handed them to me. They were completely blank, except for the children's names and dates of birth. Actually, Eliana's didn't even have a date of birth.

"This is it?" I asked incredulously. It wasn't like DSS had just met these kids. They'd been under DSS supervision for two years. Couldn't the social worker just pull this information out of a file somewhere?

Señora Gonzalez shrugged, frowning. Eliana started to whimper; Señora Gonzalez pulled a bottle out of her purse, took off the cap, and put it in the baby's mouth. She stopped crying immediately and began to suck vigorously. She didn't nestle, get comfortable the way you'd expect a baby to do while taking a bottle. Instead, she leaned back stiffly, awkwardly, her eyes darting around the room.

I took down the DSS worker's name and phone number, so that I could call to get more information about the children.

In Spanish, I asked how the children were doing, and if Señora Gonzalez had any particular concerns.

She was worried about the younger two, she told me. The baby just didn't seem right, she said. She was so small, and she didn't play or smile much, or even really cry—she just whimpered. She didn't seem to like to be held, either. Sharina was more sociable, and would play, but she didn't talk. At first Señora Gonzalez thought Sharina was just shy, but after a few days she asked Daisy and Carlos about it. They said Sharina never talked. She just pointed at what she wanted.

Daisy and Carlos were fine, she said. They were helpful and good.

There was something in Señora Gonzalez's eyes, though, when she looked at Daisy, something suspicious and tentative.

I asked if there was a problem with Daisy. Señora Gonzalez hesitated for a moment, and then said no.

I examined Daisy first. She was tentative but cooperative, taking deep breaths and opening her mouth when I asked her to, lying down, sitting up. I spoke to her in Spanish; she answered me in English.

"Let's speak Spanish," I said to her. "That way, everybody can understand." Señora Gonzalez was from the Dominican Republic and spoke very little English, and although Carlos had probably learned some from kindergarten, I doubted that Sharina and Eliana had heard much. Their mother was from Puerto Rico, a relatively recent immigrant, and spoke almost no English. Her family and her boyfriend also spoke essentially only Spanish. Señora Gonzalez knew this from the DSS worker. It was almost all she knew.

"I speak English," said Daisy. She set her shoulders squarely and tossed back her ponytail.

"I know you do," I said. "You speak it well. But I'd like to speak Spanish."

"I like English," she said. She looked past me at the wall, her expression blank and defiant at the same time.

This was about something bigger than what language we should speak, but I didn't know exactly what it was about. I didn't know what giving in, or not giving in, would mean. So I didn't do either. I spoke Spanish, and I didn't comment when she spoke English back.

Her examination was normal. She was thin, but healthy. When I examined her genitals I had Señora Gonzalez come stand near the table, in case this frightened her, but she was cooperative and calm, her hard brown eyes staring steadily at the wall. Her hymen was intact, and there was no sign of injury. Not that this proved that she hadn't been touched or injured. Sexual abuse usually doesn't leave physical signs, let alone proof.

Daisy didn't give me any signs either, no clues in her actions or reactions, and I didn't ask—not this time, when we were just meeting, and when the other children could hear. She was safe now. There was time for the unraveling, for finding out.

Carlos was next. He was more shy, more difficult. I tried to engage him, talking about the dinosaur he'd drawn. I told him I liked it.

"*Es malo,*" he said, it's bad. He crumpled up the piece of paper and threw it on the floor.

I picked it up and smoothed it out. "*¿Puedo tenerlo?*" I asked— can I have it?

He shrugged. I put it on the desk.

He was short, with brown hair that needed cutting, and a long face like Daisy's. He had a slight build that his thinness accentuated, and a voice so soft you could barely hear it.

He flinched frequently as I examined him, no matter how gentle I was, no matter how much I talked to him and told him exactly what I was going to do. He was thinner than Daisy, but he too was healthy. I looked over every inch of skin. The flinching had to mean something. There was a fading bruise on his upper right arm. I asked him what happened.

"*Me caí,*" he said—I fell. His face took on Daisy's blankness.

On the left side of his back, near his shoulder, was a small scar. It was hard to tell, but it looked like it might have been a cigarette burn. I asked him what had happened there.

He didn't answer. I asked again. He looked at the floor, and said nothing.

I started to ask the question in a different way, and then stopped. He was huddling away from me as if my questions were blows. I didn't want to do that to him. The children were going to see a psychologist soon. She was very good, and I knew that she would know how to help Carlos talk.

He looked like he wanted to cry, although I could tell he would not let himself. I wanted to change the subject, so quickly I asked what he thought of the Gonzalez family.

His face lit up immediately. *"Me gustan mucho,"* he said enthusiastically—he liked them a lot.

His enthusiasm was so immediate and genuine that I laughed. I asked him why.

"Porque me da mucha comida," he said—because I get a lot to eat.

I bit my lip. Señora Gonzalez laughed, and reached out her hand to him. He went to her, a little reluctantly. She gave him a hug; he smiled.

I picked up Sharina and put her on the exam table. She giggled. I asked her questions in Spanish about her dress, and about her doll, which she held tightly. If she could answer by nodding or shaking her head, she did; if she would have to say something to answer, she didn't answer. I asked her how old she was. She grinned, and held up two fingers.

"She doesn't talk," said Daisy.

Her voice startled me; it sounded different than it had before I examined her. It was muted, with a trace of anger. I turned to look at her; she was standing against the wall, very still, her shoulders slumped.

"Has she ever talked? Does she say anything at all?" I asked. I didn't know how to react to the change in Daisy.

"I don't remember," said Daisy. "I don't think so."

I looked in Sharina's mouth and throat and ears, which she seemed to think was great fun. I couldn't find a physical reason for her silence. She could giggle, so her vocal cords worked. She appeared to hear fine, given her responses to me and the way she turned when the baby made a noise or Carlos called to her, so deafness wasn't the reason she didn't talk. She had never learned, or she had a learning disability—or she didn't want to talk.

She had no bruises, or scars, or signs of sexual abuse, or anything else. I helped her down from the table, telling Señora Gonzalez to keep trying to get her to talk, and that we'd see what the psychologist said. Sharina went to Carlos, who was back on the floor coloring. She sat down next to him, her body up against his, and hugged her doll.

I took the baby from Señora Gonzalez, laying her on the table. I took off her clothes; she was very small for six months, and her arms and legs had almost no fat on them. She had no birth defects or signs of illness to explain her size and thinness.

I asked Señora Gonzalez if she was sure about Eliana's age, since the Medical Passport hadn't had a birth date. Maybe she was younger than six months. Señora Gonzalez said that the mother had said that the baby was six months old. She didn't know why there was no birth date. Perhaps the DSS worker had just forgotten to write it down.

"Tiene bastante apetito," said Señora Gonzalez. *"Siempre quiere comer."* The baby had a big appetite and wanted to eat all the time.

Eliana stared at me, with eyes that looked almost panicked. I examined her quickly, because her eyes disturbed me. There was a large healing bruise on the side of her head that I could see through her sparse dark hair, and there were scattered other bruises on her body. Her neurologic exam was normal, so the stiffness I'd noticed in Señora Gonzalez's arms wasn't a neurologic problem. I took down her diaper; there was a bad diaper rash.

"Ha mejorado bastante," said Señora Gonzalez when she saw me looking at the rash. *"Estaba terrible."* Apparently the rash had been much worse.

While she was with her mother, Eliana had barely been fed,

barely been changed, and from the way she was acting, it seemed like she had barely been held. She didn't nestle into Señora Gonzalez's arms because she didn't know how, because being in someone's arms was new and scary.

I dressed her again, fighting back tears.

"No es problema médico," I said to Señora Gonzalez. The baby's problem was not a medical one.

Señora Gonzalez understood. She came over and took Eliana from me, buttoning the last buttons and wrapping her in a warm blanket. The baby whimpered and squirmed, but Señora Gonzalez held her firmly and tenderly.

"Vamos a cuidarte, niñita," she said to Eliana. We are going to take care of you, little girl.

We were done. I wrote down the dates of the appointments with the psychologist, and made out appointment cards for Daisy and Carlos to go to the dentist and the eye doctor. I filled out forms for all of them to go to the lab to be checked for anemia. I said that I would call DSS to see if I could find out what immunizations the children needed, and that I would call Señora Gonzalez afterward to set up appointments for the children with me.

Señora Gonzalez listened carefully, nodding. Her graying black hair was gathered into a bun, which she smoothed absentmindedly with her hand as she listened. She was a large woman, with a soft, wrinkled face and surprising blue eyes that seemed almost to sparkle. When I was done she put the papers into a neat pile on the corner of the desk, and put Eliana into the baby carrier on the floor. She gave Daisy and Carlos their coats, which were brand-new windbreakers, and stood holding Sharina's. Sharina stood close to Carlos.

"I'll put Sharina's on," I said.

"Carlos needs to do it," said Daisy, who had moved to the corner, as far away from everyone as possible in the little room. "She only lets Carlos do things."

Señora Gonzalez knew this. She waited until Carlos had zipped his coat, and handed him Sharina's. He put it on carefully, waiting patiently for her to switch the doll from one hand to the other so that she could keep holding it as she put her coat on. He zipped it up slowly to her chin. Sharina smiled at him.

Señora Gonzalez scooped up the papers and her big black purse and then the baby carrier, adjusting it so that it hung in the crook of her arm. The baby stared up at her silently from the carrier. With her free hand Señora Gonzalez motioned to the others, easily and confidently, and like a shepherd she carefully moved them out of the room and toward the lab.

Carlos walked with a shuffle, his head down. Sharina took his hand as she crossed over the threshold of the room and held it tightly, looking up at him every few seconds as they walked down the hall. Carlos slowed down to accommodate her little steps.

Daisy hung behind. When everyone was several feet in front of her she squared her shoulders, picked up her head, and began to twirl again.

Eight

Teresa's eyes were wild.

She was trying to explain to me why she was so late—almost an hour—for her daughter's checkup. It had something to do with Lila's father. He had forgotten to tell Teresa about the appointment, or maybe it was that Teresa had forgotten; it wasn't clear to me. He had custody of Lila but he didn't take good care of her, Teresa was telling me. When he dropped her off with Teresa she was dirty and her braids were all messy. Teresa had to clean her and do her hair. And then there was a problem with the subway train. It didn't come for a long time.

I think that was what she was telling me, but her sentences were long and loose and not particularly coherent, trailing off to include things about trains in general or men in general or the finer points of braiding hair. Her voice was deep, with a touch of hoarseness that made her seem breathless. She gestured broadly with her hands, twice hitting the desk by accident.

Lila, who was three, wandered around the room inspecting things. She was tall for her age and skinny, with long brown legs that looked out of proportion to the rest of her body. She wore one of the clinic's brightly patterned hospital gowns. The yellow dress she had worn to the clinic was laid neatly at the end of the exam table. Lila's head was covered with braids; woven carefully into the braids were round white beads. She moved from the sink to the exam table to the scale, touching everything, pulling at everything. As she touched each thing, she looked over her shoulder at her mother. Teresa did not look at her.

Teresa was looking at me. Her eyes pulled at mine as she spoke.

But sometimes as she gestured, her eyes moved off to look at nothing and it was then that the sentences would trail off. In a brief moment she would pick up the sentence, stumbling with it a little until she found her pace, and then her wild eyes would be back on me.

There was another child in the room. His name was Damian, and he was nine years old. He stood in the corner sullenly, staring at his mother. He was tall, like his sister, and just as thin. His shorts and T-shirt, both blue, were dirty. His high-top sneakers had holes in the toes. Teresa brought him because she had to, she said.

"His father brought him over yesterday 'cause he goin' be busy and Damian, he get in the way or he get out on the streets and that ain't good. So I'm keeping him for a while." She looked at the boy in a distant way, her eyes running over him almost as if he were a stranger, yet there was pride in her voice.

"Do you have custody of him?"

"Nah," said Teresa blankly, looking down. "I ain't got custody of none of my kids. Lila and Damian, they's with their fathers. Ronald, he's in a foster home 'cause his father didn't want him."

"Why don't you have custody of them?" I asked.

"'Cause of the drugs," said Teresa matter-of-factly.

I was startled. I hadn't expected her to be so forthcoming with this information. I would have expected someone to at least try to hide it.

She looked up and straight at me. "You're new, aren't you?"

"Yes," I said.

"I knew it," she said. "I been coming here my whole life, so I knows everybody."

She leaned back gracefully, stretching out her long legs. I could see where Lila and Damian got their height. She was thin too, with dark, creamy brown skin. She had a gently curved nose and full lips; if she didn't look so haggard and tired, she would be beautiful. Her head was covered in a blue and yellow scarf. She wore a short-sleeved blue cotton dress, long and cut low in front, faded but flattering. I found myself staring at her arms.

She smiled at me. "I don't do needles, don't worry," she said.

I could feel myself blushing. I opened my mouth to say something, although I didn't know what it should be, and suddenly I felt something on my back. I jumped. It was Lila, taking my stethoscope off my back.

"Can I check you?" she said with a big smile. Before I could say anything she was climbing onto my lap and putting the stethoscope on.

"Lila, baby, leave the doctor alone," said Teresa.

"It's okay," I said. Lila made herself comfortable on my lap and put the stethoscope on me, listening seriously.

Although she was tall, she was so thin that she felt small in my lap. I reached around her and flipped through her chart. Damian still stood in the corner, staring at me.

"It has been a while since her last physical," I said. It had been more than a year and a half; children her age should have yearly physicals.

"I lost track," said Teresa. "Her father's supposed to be bringing her for her medical stuff, but he never do. I tries to keep track of when they gonna need physicals and stuff, her and Damian, but sometimes, sometimes I lose track."

"How much time does she spend with you?" I asked.

"Varies," said Teresa. She sat up, leaning forward to adjust a strap on her sandal. "Depends on her father, mostly. I likes to see her whenever." Her eyes wandered briefly to Lila and then came back to me.

"I got visitation once a week," she continued. "It's supposed to be what they calls 'supervised,' at his place with him around but he never wants that 'cause of his girlfriends so usually he just drop her off. Drops her off weekends a lot, and sometimes he don't come back to get her for a few days. She ain't in school, so it don't matter much. With Damian, he gotta be back with his father regular so he can go to school."

Damian shifted position and looked down at the mention of his name.

"I ain't hardly got room for them both anyway, 'cause I only gots a one-bedroom apartment, and it's real small. Lila, she sleeps in bed with me when she stays. Damian don't hardly stay over, but when he does he sleeps on the floor next to the bed. I don't like him out on the couch at night. I live on the first floor, and y'know, when you're in the projects you never can be sure if some bullet gonna come through that front window or something. Ronald, he ain't allowed to stay over. He ain't hardly allowed to visit." She didn't sound sad. She sounded resigned.

Damian shifted position again. He looked at Teresa; his dark eyes were angry. Teresa saw me looking at him and turned; quickly, he looked away and down.

"Is there anything worrying you about Lila?" I asked, trying to move the conversation back to Lila's physical.

Teresa hesitated, and frowned. "Like what?" she said.

"I don't know," I said, stumbling a little. I thought it was a self-explanatory question. "Any illnesses, or behavior problems, or anything?"

Teresa shrugged. "She's okay, I guess. Are you okay, Lila?"

Lila took off the stethoscope and smiled at her mother. "I fine," she said. She seemed for a moment like she was going to climb out of my lap and go to Teresa, but she didn't. She stayed in my lap and swung the stethoscope back and forth near the floor.

"How's her speech?" I asked. "Is she talking in sentences? Can she describe things, and ask clearly for what she wants?"

Teresa looked at Lila and frowned again. I got the feeling that the two of them didn't talk much. "She ask for what she want," said Teresa. Her eyes moved away from Lila and went off into nowhere, staying there this time.

There were more questions I would normally ask a parent, but I could see that this wasn't a normal situation, so I decided to stop. I found myself staring at Teresa again, not at her arms but at all of her—the careful knot in her scarf at the nape of her neck, the slump of her shoulders, the blankness of her expression. There was something about her that fascinated me; she was different from anyone I'd ever met before. Teresa didn't notice my stare, or if she did, she didn't say anything.

Lila delicately put the stethoscope back over my shoulder. She reached up and smoothed my hair back so that she could touch my earring, a little silver cat.

"That's pretty," she said, smiling sweetly, almost coyly.

This kind of familiarity, sitting on my lap and touching me when she had never met me, was unusual for a three-year-old. It was possible she was just a very friendly child, but it felt like there was more to her behavior than that.

"How about we check you out now, sweetie?" I said, picking her up and putting her on the exam table. I looked over at Damian, who was still in the corner. "You can sit in my chair, if you want," I said to him. Without looking at me, he slinked over and sat down, turning his body away from us and staring out the window.

I listened to Lila's heart and lungs, looked in her mouth and ears, checked her eyes, felt her stomach. She was very cooperative. She kept smiling at me, and her little hands reached up to touch me whenever she could.

"She real clean, ain't she," said Teresa.

"Yes, she is," I said.

"I cleaned her up good this morning. Her father, he don't really wash her. But I always keeps my kids clean. Least I keeps Lila clean. Damian here, he don't let me wash him no more."

Damian turned and glared at her. Teresa saw this time, but she ignored him.

"When he was a baby, though, when he was with me all the

time, I kept him so clean. Nobody could say I didn't keep my babies clean. Nobody could say that." Her voice slurred slightly on the last sentence.

I finished examining Lila. Except for her thinness, she was healthy. I lifted her down off the table. She went over to her mother, standing hesitantly in front of her. Damian got out of the chair and slinked back into the corner. I stayed standing, looking at the three of them.

"You should try to get more calories into her," I said. "Use whole milk, peanut butter, cheese, milk shakes, things like that. Offer food to her frequently."

"She is kind of skinny, huh," said Teresa. "I tries to get her to eat, but sometimes she just won't." Suddenly it seemed that Teresa's energy was gone. She looked down, her eyes no long pulling mine, and her hands lay still in her lap.

I handed Teresa the yellow dress. A little awkwardly, she took the gown off Lila and put on the dress. It was small, but it was clean and pretty. Lila tried to catch her mother's eye, smiling at her, but Teresa's concentration seemed to be taken up by the dress.

"She needs to go to the dentist, for a checkup. We like to start at her age. She should get her vision checked, too, and her hearing. And I'd like to see her back in a couple of months, to check her weight." I sat down at the desk and made out the cards for Teresa to bring to the appointment desk and handed them to her. Teresa glanced at them, nodded, and put them into her purse. I doubted the appointments would be made.

I wondered if she might be on drugs right then; I wasn't sure how I would know. In medical school we had learned about the symptoms of drug use. Sitting in the lecture hall, they seemed so clear and obvious. But sitting in the exam room, not knowing what Teresa was like normally, and realizing that lots of other things besides drug use can cause slurred speech, agitation, lethargy, and distractedness, they didn't seem clear or obvious at all.

"Where are you going after this?" I asked. I was worried that perhaps I shouldn't let the children go with her if she might be high.

"I gotta take her to the lab, right?" she said.

"No, I mean after that. After you leave the clinic." I was sure she was going to be annoyed with me for asking, or at least think it was a strange question, but her expression didn't change.

"I's taking Damian back to his father's—he lives here in the projects. Then Lila and I's going to my aunt's house up the street. Her father is going to pick her up there."

So she wasn't going to have them for very long, and she was going to be with another adult. I felt less worried.

"Who is your worker with the Department of Social Services?" I asked.

"Why?" said Teresa sharply, looking right at me. This question had a very different response than the last one.

"I—I'm just wondering who you have to help you out," I said in as friendly a tone as I could. That was more or less true, although I was also looking for ways to get more information about Teresa and her children.

"Help me out?" said Teresa. She seemed to relax, and she laughed. "I've had lots of DSS workers. They's always changing. They's like you folks here at the clinic—they never stay very long. Some helps a little, most of them don't, except to help me get into detox. They do help me with that. I forgets my worker's name, some lady even younger than you are. I goes to the office up at Dimmock."

Lila leaned against her mother's legs. Almost absentmindedly, Teresa put her arm around her. Lila smiled and leaned closer, against Teresa's breasts.

As I looked at them, I felt a sadness mixed with hope.

"Are you planning on trying to get custody of your children again?" I asked.

Teresa looked down. "I don't make plans no more," she said. "All's that happens when I make plans is that I gets disappointed."

She stood up. I handed her the form to take to the lab for Lila's blood test. Damian shot out the door, and Lila ran after him. As she turned her back to me, walking out, Teresa spoke again. She was talking more to the wall, or to nobody, than to me.

"Anyways, I ain't never getting my kids back," she said flatly. "I ain't never gonna beat the drugs."

Before I could think of anything to say, she was gone.

Nine

Who are you again?" the DSS worker asked me.

"Claire McCarthy. Dr. McCarthy," I said, as calmly as I could. "I am the Molina children's pediatrician. I have left you four messages."

"Oh," she said, and then hurriedly added, "I don't think I got any of them."

I didn't believe her, but I was so happy to actually have her on the phone that I didn't want to argue.

"I need some information about the children," I said, "and I'm hoping that you can help me."

"What kind of information?" asked the DSS worker suspiciously. Her name was Carmen Gordon. She had a trace of a Hispanic accent, and she sounded older than most of the workers I'd spoken with, maybe in her forties.

"Basic information, to start. Like Eliana's birthday. And I need medical information. I need to know what medical problems they've had, and what immunizations they've had."

She was silent for a moment. Then she said, "I don't know if I have that information."

"You don't know Eliana's birthday?" It was a facetious thing to say, but I couldn't help myself.

"I know her birthday," she said brusquely, clearly annoyed.

"So it's the medical information you're not sure you have?" I asked in the most pleasant and nonthreatening voice I could, trying to regain some ground.

"I just got this case last week. I'm still going through all the records. I'm sure the information is there. Perhaps I could get it to you in a week or two."

"I need it sooner than that. Is there anyone in your office who could go through the records and just pick out the medical information for me?"

"Dr. McCarthy, we are all very busy here." Her voice sounded strained.

"I'm sure you are," I said, feeling just as strained. I thought for a moment. "Perhaps you could just tell me where the children got their health care," I said. "Then I could call there and get the information myself."

She hesitated, and then said, "I guess I could do that." She put me on hold for a long time, and then came back with the name of the clinic.

"Also," I said, "the psychologist who is going to see them needs information about the children's background so that she can do a good evaluation."

"That information is confidential," said Mrs. Gordon.

"Of course it is," I said. "And we would respect that. But without that information, doing an evaluation would be a little like being in a minefield, and it would be hard to know what issues to concentrate on in therapy."

There was another hesitation before Mrs. Gordon said, "I'll see what I can do. Like I said, I'm just going through the records myself."

It's the bureaucracy of caring again, I thought. God forbid anything should be straightforward. I thanked her and hung up the phone.

I called the clinic where the children had gone. The secretary transferred me to the nurse, who was very sympathetic. She knew about what had happened to Eliana, as the hospital had called them when she was admitted. She put me on hold while she got the children's records.

"Wow," she said when she came back to the phone.

"What?" I asked.

"Now I remember this family. I didn't put it all together when we got the call about the baby. They'd actually only been coming here for about a year—they've moved around a lot. But you could tell they were a mess from a mile away. We called the workers a few times because we were worried—kids were behind on shots, they were dirty, Mom was rough with them, you know. The workers listened, and seemed concerned, but, well, the stuff we were calling about was never enough to take the kids away. The worker would go talk to Mom, tell her to bring the kids in, clean them up, and not to be so rough, but nothing ever got better.

"Once we filed a report of suspected abuse. One of them, let's see, it was Carlos, he had a bad bruise on his arm that made us suspicious, especially since Mom said she didn't know how it happened. This was worse than the other stuff that had worried us, so instead of just calling the worker we did an official report. DSS investigated, but suddenly Mom had a story that seemed to fit, and Carlos wouldn't talk about the bruise, so they had to drop it. They said that it didn't matter so much that they were dropping it, since Mom was under their supervision. Right."

"What about medical problems?" I asked.

"Uh, let me see. Our records aren't real complete for before they came here. We had Mom sign record requests for the other three clinics she had used, but we only got stuff from the most recent place they'd been. They had all the immunization dates, though, which was something, at least.

"Okay. Daisy was healthy. Occasional mild illness. Carlos has asthma, and Mom tended to run out of meds, so he came in pretty sick a few times. Sharina had a bunch of ear infections. Which might explain why she didn't talk, but she actually seemed to hear fine. We made an appointment for her to go to see an audiologist to check her hearing, just to be sure, but Mom didn't take her. Eliana—well, we actually only saw her twice, as a newborn and then for a cold when she was a month old. We never saw her after that, and never gave her any shots. We tried calling a bunch of times, left some messages with relatives, but she never showed up."

Eliana should have been seen at two, four, and six months for checkups and shots. She hadn't had any of those appointments.

The nurse read off the children's birthdays. The date I had for Sharina was wrong. She read off the immunization dates; Daisy was the only one who had all the shots she needed. The rest were behind.

"Thank you so much," I said. "This is incredibly helpful."

"Not really," said the nurse. "Helpful would have been getting those kids out sooner."

The next day Señora Gonzalez came to the window at Pediatrics holding Eliana, saying she had a fever and a cough and had cried all night. The other children were with her. It was a school holiday, she explained, and she had nobody to watch them.

I asked her to come in. She told Daisy and Carlos to sit in the waiting room, which was clearly visible from Pediatrics, and told Sharina to come with her. Sharina looked at Carlos and her lower lip began to quiver. Carlos looked as if he might cry too.

"She needs to be with Carlos," said Daisy sharply.

I got the feeling that Señora Gonzalez was getting used to hearing only English from Daisy.

"Ella es pequeña. Tiene que quedar conmigo," she said—Sharina was young, and had to stay with her.

Daisy glared at her. Carlos looked at her with reddened eyes that seemed ever so slightly relieved. They turned and went to the waiting room.

I led Señora Gonzalez into an exam room. "Is everything okay with Daisy?" I asked in Spanish.

"Ella es difícil," she said—she's hard. Señora Gonzalez didn't look at me as she said this, and it was clear that she didn't want to talk more about it. Sharina sat down on the floor, very near the door.

Eliana started to cough, a deep, wet cough, and then began to cry hoarsely in the baby carrier. Señora Gonzalez put it down on the exam table and picked Eliana up out of it, cradling her close.

Immediately, Eliana stopped crying. She looked up at Señora Gonzalez and relaxed, turning herself in toward and against Señora Gonzalez's body. She had learned to nestle. I smiled.

We weighed her on the baby scale in the room; she had gained a few ounces since her last visit. Señora Gonzalez laid her down on the table and I took her temperature; it was 102°F. I examined her. When I listened to her lungs I heard some faint crackles. She had pneumonia.

I gave her back to Señora Gonzalez and asked how Eliana was drinking. Oh, nothing stops her from taking her bottle, Señora Gonzalez told me with a laugh. She has a great appetite. I asked if the fever came down with Tylenol. She nodded, and looked at the clock. She was due for some now, she told me.

I explained to Señora Gonzalez that the baby had an infection in her lungs and was going to need antibiotics and close observation. I asked her if she was comfortable with this, warning her that the baby may need a lot of attention; if it was more than she could handle, given the others, I could arrange to have Eliana admitted to the hospital.

Señora Gonzalez frowned and shook her head. *"Puedo hacerlo,"* she said. *"Prefiero tenerla conmigo."* She could do it, and she preferred to have the baby with her.

I was hoping she'd say that. I was hoping she'd be willing to nurse her through the illness. Eliana needed to be held, and to matter to someone, just as much as she needed the antibiotics.

I left the room to get some more Tylenol and a shot of antibiotics so that we could begin to fight the infection right away. As I passed by the window that looked out on the waiting room, I paused to check on Daisy and Carlos.

There were a group of children playing on the small plastic slide in the middle of the rug, and a few others were chasing each other around the perimeter of the room. Daisy and Carlos were in the corner. They had turned two chairs around so that their backs were to the other children, and had pulled the chairs as close as possible. They sat there together, arms touching. It was noisy in the waiting room, but I could hear that they were singing. It was a song I'd never heard before, a repetitive, plaintive, almost haunting song.

It was more than a week before Mrs. Gordon from DSS called me again, and she didn't have much to offer. She told me that there had been a suspicion of sexual abuse of Daisy that hadn't been proved, that the mother had a long history of drug abuse, and that they thought that Carlos had probably been physically abused. I asked if there were any more details she could give me; she hesitated and said again that it was confidential.

I called her supervisor, a soft-spoken man who sounded younger than she. I explained again how important the information was. He listened without commenting and said that he would see what he could do.

A few days later, a big manila envelope arrived in the mail for me. Inside it was a pile of records from DSS about the children. They were poor quality photocopies of handwritten notes, social workers' reports, and other seemingly random documentation. There was no cover letter, and they were in no particular order. The only summary I could find was stuck in the middle and outdated. It took me quite a while just to put things into a readable order.

They were scattered puzzle pieces, pockets of time, incomplete—but, nonetheless, shocking. I had been told that DSS became involved at the time of Sharina's birth, but actually they had been involved earlier, when Daisy was four and Carlos was two. Daisy told a preschool teacher that her mother's boyfriend had been "touching her 'down there,'" and the teacher filed a report of suspected sexual abuse. Daisy was seen by a psychologist, and she told him that this boyfriend frequently came into her bed and fondled her. The psychologist was impressed by the details that Daisy was able to provide, and told DSS that he believed her story. The boyfriend, who had a history of drug possession and trafficking charges, was arrested. His lawyer disputed Daisy's story, saying there was no physical evidence, and that Daisy had made everything up. Daisy's mother agreed with the boyfriend and his lawyer, saying that Daisy watched a lot of television and had a very active imagination. Despite the psychologist's report and the pediatrician's attempts to explain that fondling wouldn't necessarily leave physical evidence, the molestation charges were dropped.

DSS followed the family for about nine months after that. The mother broke up with the boyfriend, and went into drug treatment. The apartment was always relatively clean and stocked with food when the worker came to visit, and the children seemed well cared for, so DSS closed the case. There was a comment, though, scribbled at the bottom of a page by the worker, like an afterthought, that chilled me.

"Daisy's teacher reports that since the molestation charges were dropped Daisy has become withdrawn."

The image of Daisy on the day I met her, in the corner of the exam room, as far from everyone as possible, flashed into my mind. Of course Daisy withdrew, I thought. I would too, if I couldn't trust people to take care of me.

The next documentation was dated two years later, when Sharina was born and tested positive for cocaine. The hospital filed a report, and DSS became involved again. The notes from that investigation said that the mother had dropped out of the drug treatment program shortly after the previous case with DSS was closed, and since then had been using drugs intermittently. Daisy was six, and had missed most of first grade. Carlos was four. The mother hadn't enrolled him in preschool because, she said, she didn't have to and the preschool teachers were too nosy. She hadn't brought him to the pediatrician since the previous case was closed, either. The boyfriend who had been accused of molesting Daisy was back—he was Sharina's father.

The worker doing the investigation asked Daisy if the boyfriend had touched her or otherwise made her uncomfortable. The first two times she was asked she wouldn't answer. The third time, she said no.

The mother was described as disorganized and unkempt. The worker said that she showed only rare signs of affection for the children. When the worker questioned the mother about her own family the mother said that her father had abandoned them when she was a baby, and that her mother was an alcoholic.

The worker noticed that the mother had bruises on her face, and asked about them. The mother said that the bruises were from a fall, but refused to give any details about the fall; from her secretiveness and the type of bruising, the worker suspected that she may have been beaten—but when asked this directly, the mother denied it.

As I read this part, I realized that I had never actually had any feelings or thoughts about the mother besides anger. She was faceless evil to me. I was still angry, but I realized how little I knew about her and about her prisons of addiction and violence. Nothing could make what she did excusable, but people are not so simple as wrong and right. They are intrinsically complicated, and pain is very powerful.

The family was deemed to be at significant risk, and a "service plan" was made involving immediate drug treatment for the mother, psychological treatment for the children, and close supervision of the family.

What happened after that was a little unclear from the records. There was a lot of turnover in the workers—there appeared to be at least three involved with the family. Each time the worker changed, it looked like there was a transition period where supervision and enforcement lagged while the worker got to know the family. The mother was in and out of treatment—she'd complain about the program she was in at the time, drop out, be threatened with the loss of her children, go back in, over and over again. The psychological treatment for the children never happened—the mother made appointments but never went, saying she had no transportation, the weather was bad, the baby was sick, or something else. The family had no phone and seemed to be out of the apartment frequently, making close supervision difficult.

How common this must be, I thought. I could imagine each little incident, each missed appointment, or each time when nobody answered the door. Each time, it must have been frustrating, but it probably didn't seem like a big deal. It was only in looking back, after Eliana was beaten so badly, that the sheer number of these incidents and their meaning became clear. I wondered how many other families were so hard to supervise closely, and how many children in those families would subsequently be hurt—or die.

There wasn't much about Carlos. His kindergarten teacher filed a report because of bruising on his back. He wouldn't tell her how it happened. The report was "screened out" because DSS was already involved with the family. There was no mention of Sharina's lack of speech. Apparently none of the children ever talked when the workers came to visit.

"The children are very quiet at visits," one of them wrote. "It is hard to tell if they are just shy, or scared."

People at DSS seemed genuinely concerned about the family, especially when Eliana was born and tested positive for cocaine. There was mention of discussions about removing the children from the home, but it seemed as if each time they began to discuss it seriously the mother would go back into drug treatment and things would seem better with the family and the decision would be postponed. It is easy now to look back and say that they should have done things differently. But it is clear that DSS had tried very hard to help the family.

I ran through the pile of papers, looking at the dates. Each entry was separated by a few weeks or months. In between those entries, in between those visits and the times that people were talking about this family, were days and days. Morning after morning for those children of waking up to the same home, the same mother high on drugs, the same abusive boyfriend, the same hunger and fear. It must have been eternity, and eternity again, for them.

I brought the records to the psychologist's office and sat while she looked through them. Sara Daviles was in her early thirties, small and athletic, with short dark hair, big earrings, and horn-rimmed glasses. She had a confident, to-the-point manner, yet at the same time her warmth had a comforting, reassuring effect on people around her.

"None of this suprises me," she said. "And I'll bet there's much more we'll never find out."

She looked up at me. "I don't think Daisy will ever tell me anything. The two times I've met with her, once with Carlos and Sharina and once alone, she just sat there and glared at me. Carlos wouldn't say anything either when Daisy was in the room, but when I was alone with him he did talk a little."

She pulled out a file from her cabinet and looked at her notes. "The stuff he says is heartbreaking. They were afraid of the boyfriend because he beat them and their mother frequently, so they used to hide, especially evenings and weekends when he was likely to come over. They'd all hide under the bed, or in the closet, or in the bathtub with the curtain drawn, changing the place all the time, trying to be really quiet so he wouldn't think to look for them. They'd bring Sharina in with them. They told her she had to be very quiet. They tried bringing Eliana too, but they couldn't stop her from crying so they had to leave her out in her crib."

She shook her head. "Carlos feels responsible for what happened to Eliana. He thinks that they should have brought her with them and found a way to stop her from crying."

"He's only six," I said. "He wasn't responsible."

"You and I know that," said Sara, "but he doesn't. And he's angry with himself for not fighting the boyfriend more, but he was afraid. Once Daisy bit the boyfriend when he tried to touch her—sounded like sexually, from the little Carlos said—and the boyfriend beat her pretty badly. Carlos said that his mother kept Daisy in the apartment until the bruises were gone."

She closed the file and put it back into the file cabinet. "I asked him what he wanted to be when he grew up, and he said in this weird, matter-of-fact way that he wasn't going to grow up."

"Did he say why?" I asked.

"I asked him," said Sara. "He said that he didn't want to."

Eliana was very sick for a few days with the pneumonia, but recovered steadily after that. When she was well I had Señora Gonzalez bring the children in for their immunizations.

As I walked into the exam room, Daisy jumped down off the exam table and stood in front of me. She still moved with the deftness of a dancer, but there was a forcefulness to her movements that had not been there before.

"You're not doing anything to me today," she said.

"No, I'm not," I said. "You've had all your shots."

"You're going to hurt my brother and sisters," she said. Her voice was as strong and defiant as the stance she had taken: legs straight, hands on hips. Her eyes sparkled as they glared at me, and she tossed her long hair over her shoulder. Her hair had become shiny and smooth since being in foster care, and her cheeks had more color.

"*Daisy, por favor,*" said Señora Gonzalez, giving her a look of annoyance and frustration. She apologized to me. "*Lo siento, doctora.*"

"I'm not sorry," said Daisy. "It's true, you are going to hurt them."

"Shots do hurt a little," I said. "But they're quick."

Carlos brought his knees up to his chin, huddling in the chair. Sharina looked at him and began to cry.

"*Ven, Sharina,*" said Señora Gonzalez, motioning for Sharina to come to her. She moved Eliana, who was sitting in her lap, onto one knee and lifted Sharina onto the other. Eliana grabbed Sharina's hospital gown and giggled. Sharina smiled, wiped her tears, and leaned back against Señora Gonzalez's breast.

"*Eliana parece bastante mejor,*" I said—Eliana looks much better. Señora Gonzalez smiled and nodded. Eliana really did look better, not just from the pneumonia but in general. She had gained weight, her eyes were brighter, she was obviously happy, and she had begun to sit up by herself. In one short month she was a different baby.

"*¿Quién primero?*" I asked.

"*La más pequeña,*" said Señora Gonzalez, pointing to Eliana as the one she wanted to do first. She stood up with the two girls and put Sharina down on the chair, giving her a kiss on the head as she did so. She brought the baby to the table and laid her down. I gave her the shots she needed as quickly as I could. She screamed, but stopped almost immediately when Señora Gonzalez picked her up and hugged her.

I turned to Sharina. Her eyes had grown huge upon seeing the needles. Señora Gonzalez put Eliana down on the exam table and motioned to Daisy to come hold on to the baby there so she wouldn't fall off. Daisy stood against the wall, her arms folded in front of her, and shook her head.

"*Por favor,*" said Señora Gonzalez. Her voice was stern. Señora Gonzalez was not a stern woman; it was clear that she and Daisy argued a lot.

"No," said Daisy.

"Please, Daisy," I said. "We need your help, so that Señora Gonzalez can hold Sharina. Just for a second. You don't need to hold Eliana, just put your hand on her so that she doesn't fall."

Daisy came forward sullenly and picked Eliana up off the table. She put Eliana on her hip, as easily and naturally as an experienced mother.

Señora Gonzalez picked up Sharina and brought her to the table. Sharina began to scream and kick, trying to get away. Señora Gonzalez tried to calm her, but Sharina would not be calmed. She reached out her tiny hand toward Carlos, who had been on the edge of his chair ever since she started to scream. He ran to her and took her hand; she stopped screaming.

I pulled a chair close to the table and had Señora Gonzalez sit in it, holding Sharina. I had Carlos stand close by, holding Sharina's hand, and I gave her the shots. When I was done Carlos picked her up and hugged her, holding her very tight, until she stopped crying. Señora Gonzalez smiled at him, and whispered softly in his ear, "*Qué buen hermano,*" what a good brother.

As soon as Sharina was out of Señora Gonzalez's lap, Daisy handed Eliana to her and went back to the wall. I was about to go look for someone to help hold Carlos, rather than fight with Daisy again, when he put Sharina down on the chair and climbed up slowly onto the table himself.

"I ready," he said.

"Are you sure?" I asked.

He nodded, closed his eyes, and stiffened.

"It's just shots, to keep you healthy. It's not because you did anything bad, you do know that, don't you?" I said. He didn't respond.

I trembled a little, incredibly uncomfortable being this person he had made me into. I gave him his two shots. He didn't cry; he didn't even flinch. When I was done he just sat there, as if waiting for more.

"Oh, honey," I said, and I put my arms around him.

Ten

Home became my refuge, my place to let go a bit, to forget a bit. In Mark's arms everything felt softer and more possible, and Michaela had a lovely way of reminding me that although there was a lot of badness in the world, there was a lot of goodness in it too. And about six months after going to work at Martha Eliot I had something else to take my mind off my work: I was pregnant again.

The second time around, I knew what pregnancy would bring and when. I could predict what times of day I would be tired, what would make me nauseated, and when my belly would outgrow my clothes. I knew when what I was feeling was baby kicks and not gas. I knew what real contractions felt like, so I could differentiate them from the common "practice" ones of pregnancy. I knew the comfortable sleeping positions, and that I should just go ahead and buy bigger sneakers.

I had everything all ready. I had the bigger bras and the maternity clothes. My first was born in the winter and my second was due in the summer, so I did have to do some shopping—but I knew which brands were best, and that I shouldn't buy those big elastic waist things because they inevitably slipped off or became uncomfortable toward the end of the pregnancy. I had baby clothes, bedsheets, cloth diapers, tiny washcloths, and all the other assorted necessary accompaniments of babydom.

But it wasn't all easier, and it certainly wasn't the same. Being pregnant with my second was a very different experience from being pregnant with my first.

When I was pregnant with Michaela I was a pediatric resident, and this was hard. I was working long hours in the hospital— ten- to twelve-hour days with frequent thirty-six-hour shifts as well. The residency program cut me remarkably little slack; I was expected to do the same work as all the other residents, no matter how I felt. This attitude surprised me initially; after all, I was working in a children's hospital, where you'd think they would be supportive of mothers-to-be. But residents were thought of as drones more than as actual people, expected to get the work done and not have needs. And although some of the other residents were supportive and helped ease my workload, many of them were so stressed and overworked that they were unwilling to take on any more.

During the end of my ninth month, I spent my days doing an elective rotation at a private pediatrician's office, which was fairly low-key, but I spent every fourth night as the senior resident in the intensive care unit. My belly had gotten so big at that point with my ten-pound daughter inside that walking had become uncomfortable, so I sat in a chair with wheels and pushed myself backward from bed space to bed space. The intensive care unit senior is also officially the "code team leader," expected to rush to any "Code Blue" (somebody trying to die) in the hospital and be in charge. I was lucky that there was only one Code Blue while I was on call that month, and that it was near the intensive care unit, because I couldn't exactly rush very well.

But outside of the hospital, my time was my own. Granted, there wasn't all that much of it, but I could spend it as I wished. I could sleep if I was tired. I could sit on the couch with my feet up and read a book. I could cook a nice meal for Mark and me—or not cook at all, if cooking made me nauseated that day. And if I felt really awful, I could call in sick from work.

The problem with the second pregnancy was that I couldn't call in sick from parenthood.

★ ★ ★

For a few days after the little strip on the pregnancy test turned blue, I felt nothing but happiness. I watched families with more than one child and was excited at the thought of being like them, at the thought of having "kids." Somehow, the plural sounded tremendously different from the singular, and connoted to me a whole different life. I daydreamed about introducing Michaela to her new sibling, about pushing them on the swings at the park, or about the four of us sitting on the couch reading a story.

The pregnancy, however, was nowhere near so idyllic. I couldn't sit or sleep when I needed to, for there was a child to care for, a child who woke up at five in the morning and was in an active, exploratory phase of her development. It didn't matter if I was exhausted; I still had to play with Michaela and watch her constantly, to be sure she wasn't doing things like climbing on furniture, putting rocks in her mouth, or torturing the cats. She was slow to walk, and for this I was grateful; it is easier to catch a crawling child than a running one. And it didn't matter how much strong smells, or cooking, nauseated me. Her poopy diapers needed to be changed, and she had to be fed. Any free time during Michaela's naps I spent napping myself, for I was exhausted. There was no part of my time that was mine; all of it belonged to Michaela or to the pregnancy.

During my pregnancy with Michaela, the growth in my belly and breasts (and hips and thighs) brought something pretty close to panic. For years, I had exercised and dieted and otherwise ensured that I stayed thin, and it was hard to imagine my distorted body ever getting thin again. But after going through labor, after a child actually emerged from my body, getting thin again didn't matter so much. For the first time in my life, I realized that my body was intrinsically beautiful, separate from whether it was fat or thin, separate from anything it looked like, because of what it could do. It could walk, dance, run, climb—and give birth to another human being.

So when I got pregnant again, I thought that it would be easy to deal with the body changes. I thought I would be calm and peaceful about it all. To some extent, this was true; I didn't panic. But as I watched all those parts of me get big again, I felt a little sad. Like so much of my life, my body seemed no longer mine. It belonged to Michaela and this child inside me and any other child we might have.

The feeling of loss of mine-ness was reinforced at the clinic, for the pregnancy definitely belonged to everyone there. This wasn't particular to my pregnancy, of course. Our lives are very public there, and very shared.

The close quarters had a lot to do with it. Most of our work when we weren't physically with patients was carried out in the secretaries' area, which was about six feet by six feet, or in the staff room, which was about ten by ten. This was where we discussed patients, made phone calls, wrote in charts, and otherwise carried out the business of patient care. On a busy day there could easily be two doctors, a nurse practitioner, three nurses, two nursing assistants, and two secretaries sharing these spaces. It's rare that everyone was in the room at once, of course, but there were moments when a lot of us were. Add to that the staff from other parts of the clinic who stopped by on patient matters or to socialize, as well as the med students and nursing students who sometimes rotated through, and drug company reps and other visitors, and soon it became like a sardine can. It is hard to find privacy in a sardine can; every smile, every conversation, every everything was noticed. Personalities became magnified, and emotions were hard to contain within one person; good moods and bad moods spread.

Most of the people who work at the clinic are women, which adds another dimension to the noticing. In general, it is easier to hide things from men. Men are more likely to accept an explanation, no matter how improbable, and are less likely to watch for or pick up on the subtle nuances of behavior that can tell so much. Women more often realize the significance of how things are said, like the tone of voice in the "Hello" or "I'm fine," or the things left unsaid. They are more likely to read the anger in the way a back is turned or the sadness in shoulders slightly slumped.

The secrets gleaned or suspected quickly spread throughout the clinic, for gossip is rampant. One becomes used to this, because there is simply no choice. It cannot be fought or changed.

What saves the scrutiny from becoming unbearable in Pediatrics is that the people who work there are without exception good at heart. They may talk about you behind your back, but they will fight for you, too, and give generously of whatever they have. There is genuine interest and concern as our stories are shared. We are, truly, like family.

So I wasn't really surprised when people at the clinic were full of questions and advice about my pregnancy. Every moment and inch of it was discussed, worried about, made fun of, and otherwise incorporated into the daily life of the clinic. My belly was everyone's property; people would tap it as they passed me in the hall, saying "Hello, baby," and would put both hands on it to assess size or feel for kicks while I was on the phone. Rarely did anyone ask permission before they touched me, and soon it no longer occurred to me that they should.

When I was four and a half months pregnant I had an ultrasound, which showed that I was carrying a very normal baby boy.

The technician showed us his face in profile. He looked so perfect, so lovely, and as we watched he brought his hand up to his face, as if to suck his thumb. Mark and I both laughed. The technician moved the probe, and we could see his tiny feet with all their toes. "Look, he's kicking!" she said. She didn't have to tell me, for I'd felt it, but watching it happen at the same time as I felt it was surreal. The fact of this baby hit me. Up until that moment, I'd just felt pregnant, in the sense of having a condition. But suddenly I was incredibly aware that inside me was a little boy—Michaela's brother, Mark's son, my son.

In the car on the way home I was quiet, staring out the window. I pictured myself holding this little boy in my arms instead of in my belly. I wondered how I would manage if he and Michaela were crying at the same time. I wondered what kind of baby he would be, what kind of child, what kind of man. I wondered how I would cook dinner with two children underfoot, how I would be able to watch both at the park, whether I'd be able to keep up with the laundry. I wondered if having two would make me a different mother.

The mothers at the clinic were just as full of questions and advice as the staff. They asked me how I was feeling, all the time. They told me about teas I could prepare to help with the nausea. They talked about the aches and pains and problems they'd had with their pregnancies and deliveries, I suppose in the spirit of commiseration, although it didn't always make me feel better.

Their hands were all over my belly, too, commenting on its shape and size, on the fact that I was carrying high. A couple of weeks after the ultrasound an eight-year-old girl I was giving a checkup to put her hands on my belly, inspected it from both sides, and announced with remarkable certainty that I was having a boy.

"You're right," I said, dumbfounded.

"She always is," said her mother.

The mothers talked about their own transitions into having more than one child, and here I listened closely. They talked about how it was hard at the beginning, especially when the children were close in age, as mine would be, but that I shouldn't get disheartened because it gets better with time. They told me the ways they'd found to keep the older child occupied while they fed the baby, and about how it was best to cook and do housework in the morning because in the afternoon everybody got tired and nothing got done. They told me to go be with other mothers, for my own support and for help in watching and amusing the older child. They said that my second child would probably bring unexpected challenges, for all children are different. But with the second, they said, you have more confidence, which makes it easier. They enjoyed telling me these things and everything else; their eyes would be bright and they'd gesture and laugh. Sometimes I'd have to cut them off so that we could talk about the child they'd brought to see me.

For a while, I wondered how the mothers knew I needed help, knew how much I didn't know. I wondered if they thought that I was incompetent or inept. But they weren't treating me that way, and slowly I realized that the mothers knew that the only way to learn certain things was to live them—or learn from someone who has lived them.

It was an exchange, a new way of seeing my relationships with patients and families, a way that I liked. They were doing more than giving me tips. They were teaching me that we all have something to teach each other.

Zachary Telles Brown was born on August 15, 1992. My doctor induced my labor three weeks before my due date because he was worried about some bleeding I was having. It was only slight bleeding, but he was concerned there might be a tear in the placenta that the ultrasound hadn't picked up, and he didn't want to take any chances. I didn't mind having the baby early, not just because of the bleeding but because the ninth month of pregnancy is not particularly comfortable, especially in August, and I was happy to have it over with.

Having the baby early meant that I worked at the clinic until the very end, until the Friday before the Saturday of the scheduled induction. It was an ordinary Friday: I saw patients, wrote in charts, made the usual phone calls, read the usual mail. And yet it wasn't ordinary at all. It was just a day, only hours, before I was to have a baby. Nothing was different, but everything was about to be. I looked at the babies I saw that day and thought: tomorrow I will have a new one of my own. It was like having a crystal ball.

It was an easier labor than I had with Michaela, mostly because Zachary weighed seven pounds instead of ten. The doctor started the induction at around eleven in the morning, and by seven that evening I had pushed out a wet, screaming baby boy.

He was so different from his sister, from the very start. She had been fat and compact at birth; he was long and skinny. She had lots of dark hair; he was completely bald. She fussed a lot; after his initial screaming, Zachary was content to be in my arms, staring at this weird new world. The difference in his presence caught me by surprise. He was, indeed, uncharted territory.

Mark had saved up vacation time and sick leave, and was home with me for a month after Zack's birth. Besides helping with cooking and housework, what he mostly did was take care of and play with Michaela, so that I could rest and breast-feed and otherwise take care of the baby. Having him home allowed us to ease into the juggling act of having two children; we could each try out strategies for handling both at once, and if they didn't work, we could go back to the one-on-one tactic.

I found that if I read stories to Michaela while I breast-fed she wouldn't wander off, and I wouldn't have to keep interrupting the feeding to go find her. We discovered that gates in doorways helped to keep her nearby when our hands were tied up with the baby. Organization was key: at night I'd lay out clothes, grind coffee, and otherwise plan for the morning, and in the morning I'd chop vegetables for dinner, pack the diaper bag, do any absolutely necessary chore, and plan for the day. The mothers at the clinic were right: in the afternoon everybody did get tired and nothing got done. It didn't matter how big the dust bunnies or piles of unfolded laundry were—by three o'clock I was either trying to calm a screaming child or collapsed on the couch, and from then until bedtime we were in pure survival mode.

The mothers at the clinic were right about lots of things, I realized, as I found myself putting more and more of their advice to use. There are some parts of parenting that are particular to culture, place, socioeconomic class. But most of its joys and struggles and details are universal.

The first day Mark went back to work I let Michaela watch all the videos she wanted, and managed to amuse her without taking her anywhere. There were a couple of crises when the two of them screamed for me at the same time (Michaela won both times—she screamed louder and had greater escalation potential, so I took care of her first), but besides that, the day was uneventful and even pleasant. The next day was warm and sunny and it seemed unfair to keep Michaela inside so, emboldened with the success of my first day alone, I decided to take the two of them to the park. It was fenced in, after all; how hard could it be? So I packed the diaper bag, put the two of them into our new double stroller, and off we went.

The double stroller turned out to be unwieldy and hard to push, and by the time I reached the park I was out of breath. I propped open the gate, which opened into the sandpit, and with tremendous effort pushed the stroller through the sand. There were a few mothers and children playing nearby with buckets and shovels. One of the mothers, a woman in her twenties with very long brown hair whose little boy looked about Michaela's age, smiled at me and said hello. She looked familiar; I vaguely remembered chatting with her a few months before. I nodded to her, too intent on trying to get the stroller out of the sandpit to start a conversation.

I made it over to a bench in the shade that was near Michaela's favorite play area. As soon as the stroller stopped moving, Zack started to scream. I looked at my watch; he was due to be fed. Michaela started to fuss, too, wanting to be let out to go play.

"Okay, you can go play," I said as I lifted her out. "But stay over here, so that Mommy can see you."

She did, for a few moments. But just as I got myself comfortable on the bench, found a way to open my shirt without my breast being in full view, and Zachary had started sucking, she ran toward the sandpit. I called to her to come back, but she kept going, with the willfull determination so typical of a nineteen-month-old. I took Zack off my breast, rearranged my bra and shirt, and ran after her, carrying her back in one arm and the screaming baby in the other.

"Now, please, Michaela, stay over here. Mommy needs to feed the baby."

Michaela nodded solemnly, and went to go play on the little slides in front of us. I went back to the bench, and tried again to feed Zack. As soon as I had him settled and nursing, I looked up; Michaela was running away again.

I jumped up and took Zack off my breast again; he started to scream again. Barely covering myself, I started after Michaela.

As I got to the sandpit, the mother with the long brown hair stood up and came to me. She reached out her hand and touched my shoulder.

"I'll watch her," she said. "I'm down here anyway. You feed the baby."

She handed a pail and shovel to Michaela, who promptly sat down in the sand and started digging.

In the moment of that small, simple kindness I understood what everyone at the clinic had been trying to show me: that we are not meant to parent alone. We are meant to be part of a community, where hands come out to guide us and help hold our children, where voices chime and mingle with ours, teaching us, comforting us. Our children are meant to grow up under many watchful eyes, and to have the love and encouragement of many.

Eleven

The mother brought the boy to "the window." It wasn't exactly a window, just a half wall, a counter, that separated the secretaries' area of Pediatrics from the lobby. This was where the families came with their pink registration slips to give to the secretary when they had appointments and where they came to ask to be seen when they didn't have appointments. They'd pick the children up to show us their rashes and cuts, or hear their coughs, or feel their skin hot with fever. We ask people to call for appointments instead of just showing up so that we can schedule appropriately, and most do, but every day there are the "walk-ins." This happens in all pediatric practices, I imagine, but in our practice the number of walk-ins can get overwhelming. Some say they don't have a phone, or were too worried to wait for the call back, or were at the clinic for another appointment and thought they'd show us the child—but most have no particular excuse. There was something wrong with their child, so they came. And although it drives us crazy and causes scheduling nightmares, their simple, direct response to the problem is hard to argue with.

The boy was about three years old; his head was well below the top of the half wall. His mother, a slender, small, African-American woman, hoisted him up on her hip for us to see. On her other hip was a baby girl, about nine months old.

"I think his asthma is acting up," said the mother. "I ran out of medicine."

Elisa, the other secretary, turned to me. I was on "follow-up" that morning of my first day back, catching up on patients, going through mail and otherwise reorganizing, not seeing patients until the afternoon. I happened to be standing there because I had come to ask Elisa a scheduling question. It is officially the job of the nurse or the doctor doing Triage to check on the patients at the window. But at Martha Eliot job descriptions blur, and proximity can rule. Whoever is near the phone when it rings answers it. Whoever is standing in the way of the lab tech coming with the abnormal result takes care of it. And whoever is standing near the window when the patient needs to be looked at looks at the patient.

The boy had a winter coat on, so I couldn't see his chest, but I could tell that he was having some trouble breathing: his shoulders moved up and down quickly, and he looked pale and uncomfortable. I unzipped his coat and snuck my stethoscope under his shirt in the back to listen to his breathing. He was wheezing badly.

I motioned the mother through the swinging doors and into one of the exam rooms; she came in, still carrying both children. Alison followed them in and began talking to the mother as she took the boy from her, put him on the exam table, and began to get his coat and shirt off so we could see and listen to his chest. The mother put the baby down on the chair and helped Alison, answering her questions.

"I should have called before to get some more medicine, but he's been doing okay these days. But then yesterday when I picked him up from day care he was getting a cold, and by early this morning he was wheezing. I stayed home from work but my husband couldn't and he had to take the car. I was getting worried, waiting for my sister to drive me over. I tried bringing him in the bathroom and turning on the shower, like you do with the croup, but that didn't help much."

"No," said Alison, "it wouldn't. He needs medicine." She wrote down his usual medicine and dose on the Triage sheet Elisa had given her, and counted his heart rate and respirations with her stethoscope. She stuck a thermometer under his arm to check his temperature; he didn't have a fever. She moved with quick, easy expertise; she had done this hundreds of times. She knew exactly what to ask and how to ask it; she knew what to do and how to do it gently and well. She knew the families, also, which was so very important; knowing the context of what people say is crucial to knowing what they really mean.

Alison enjoyed herself, too. Not that she didn't complain or get into bad moods, because she did—but it was inevitable, being as open to people and aware of them as she was; things didn't just slide off her as they would off someone who didn't care so much. But she laughed a lot, with patients and with us, and there was something about her that shone. The children always seemed to find their way into her arms.

The boy sat small and scared on the table. The muscles of his chest pulled in tightly around his ribs with each breath as he struggled to get enough air in and out. His black, curly hair was cut close to his head; he had heavy-lidded eyes that stared at Alison.

I stayed at the threshold of the room, waiting to see if Alison needed anything, as the pediatrician doing Triage was busy with another patient. Alison got out the oxygen tank, mask, and tubing for an aerosol treatment. She looked up at me as she measured the dose of the medication; I nodded.

The boy started to cry as Alison put the mask on. Most kids don't like masks, but they are the best way to make sure that most of the medicated mist goes into the child instead of all over the room. The mother climbed up on the table and put him into her lap; he leaned back against her and stopped crying. I turned to leave and nearly tripped over the baby, who had climbed out of the chair and was crawling toward the door.

"Shauna!" said the mother. I picked the baby up, but as soon as the mother's arms reached out for her, the boy began to cry again. He clearly wanted his mother all to himself. There was no stroller to strap the baby into, and she obviously wasn't going to stay in the chair if I put her there. Sarah and Marta were busy, and although the secretaries sometimes held babies while they did their work, it wasn't exactly the best way to get things done.

I put Shauna on my hip. "I'll hold her for a while," I said. The mother smiled gratefully and apologetically.

Actually, having a baby on my hip felt very comfortable on that first day back from maternity leave, more comfortable than listening to lungs or checking medication doses. I wove my way through the hallway, around a mother holding a child impatiently outside an exam room, past Marta stamping up lab forms, around two children pestering Elisa for stickers. Elisa was calmly and firmly telling them in Spanish that the stickers were only for the children who had appointments. She was only twenty-two years old, but she had so much confidence that she seemed older. I had yet to see her flustered, which was impressive given how crazy things could get.

I went back to the staff room, where I sat down next to the pile of patients' charts that I'd gathered, and put the baby on my lap. She pulled at my stethoscope; I took it off and gave it to her to play with.

Dr. Reilly, the pediatrician doing Triage, was intently checking lab results on the computer. A fair-haired, matter-of-fact woman in her forties, she had been at the clinic for years and knew so much about pediatrics and the details of inner-city life that it intimidated me. Helen was on the phone with a mother, talking in Spanish about how to bring down a fever, carefully repeating each instruction several times. Betty was sorting the day's mail into people's boxes, softly mumbling to herself as she always did. Nobody said anything about Shauna. Winter is a busy time in the clinic, and people are less chatty. Besides, we have babies in the staff room all the time, so there was nothing particularly remarkable about it.

I'd expected more talk in general, at least about my maternity leave. I'd been given a big welcome when I first arrived that morning, with lots of hugs, and the pictures I'd brought of Zachary were passed around and scrutinized with genuine interest. But then it was time to get to work; the pictures were handed back to me and everyone scattered to their places and their tasks.

Not that my feelings were really hurt. I wanted the routines and the rhythms to be the same. It was nice to slip back into the clinic and the person I was there, like slipping into a comfortable old shoe. I'd missed the work of being a doctor, seeing patients and thinking about ways to solve, or at least help, their problems. And I'd missed the clinic, very much.

It didn't feel like anything had changed. The staff room certainly hadn't; it was just as crowded and cluttered. Some of the same random pieces of paper were still there from four months ago, bits of people's mail that they meant to do something with or throw out but that ended up stuck between textbooks or under a pile of manila folders. Every once in a while Sarah would get fed up with the room and clean it, but even then the problem of the random pieces of paper persisted, because Sarah was never sure if they were important and the person whom they belonged to invariably wasn't working that day. So she would put them somewhere neatly, amid the binders and reference materials, and the clutter would grow.

I opened the chart on the top of my pile: a child with lead poisoning who had been missing appointments before I left for my leave. I wanted to find out what had happened while I was gone, and to make sure he had a follow-up appointment. Looking through the chart, I saw that he had been seen once a couple of months before, and his lead level had come down slightly. He needed another appointment as soon as possible. I put the chart aside to wait until Dr. Reilly was done on the computer, so that I could check to see if the appointment had been made.

Shauna swung the stethoscope up in the air and hit me on the head.

"No, sweetie. You don't play with it like that," I said.

She frowned at me and did it again. I took it away from her; she frowned more deeply and started grabbing the charts.

"No way, little girl. Let's do something else," I said, reaching for my pile of mail. I handed her an advertisement from a pharmaceutical company and started reading a letter from a cardiologist about one of my patients. Shauna threw the advertisement on the floor and grabbed my letter.

"Okay, this isn't going to work." I picked her up and went back out into the hallway. There were now three mothers at the window and the rack where charts of children waiting to be seen were kept was filling. I looked in on Shauna's brother; he was starting his second treatment, curled up in his mother's arms. I moved Shauna to my other hip and went back down the hallway, looking for a toy.

"*¡Doctora McCarthy!*" I heard someone say, and turned to see a woman motioning to me from one of the exam rooms. "*¿Como está Ud.?*"

It was Señora Figueroa, one of my favorite mothers, a gentle, soft-spoken woman from Guatemala who had three daughters. They were all there, sitting together on the exam table. They were four, six, and eight, all as lovely and soft-spoken as their mother. They wore matching red dresses that were clean and pressed, and their hair was carefully braided. I'd never seen them anything but perfectly dressed, even when one was sick and had kept Señora Figueroa up all night.

Señora Figueroa's husband worked at a hotel as a janitor, and in the evenings she cleaned offices. They worked long hours and made very little money, but they were proud—proud of their jobs, proud of their tiny apartment, proud of their daughters. Poverty touched them less than it did other people, perhaps because they didn't consider themselves poor. They had a place to live, food on the table, and clothes for their children; they considered themselves lucky. They believed in themselves as people and as a family, something that I was finding could be a real obstacle for others.

I went over to talk to her but the youngest daughter, who was at the clinic because of diarrhea, suddenly said that she had to go to the bathroom, so Señora Figueroa apologized sweetly to me and whisked her off.

It was good to see her, to know that she and her daughters were okay and were the same. There were so many people I was anxious to hear about and see. It had only been four months, but so much can happen in four months.

That is what makes primary care so different from other kinds of medicine: getting to know all about people, and knowing them over time. As I see families again and again, I wonder and worry about what will happen next for them. Will the illness get better? Will they keep their jobs? Will they find a place to live? Will those brothers stop fighting, and will that sister stop being so jealous of the baby? Will the landlord do something about the cockroaches? Will the children be able to go to college? Is there anything more I can do?

Lives are an unnerving mix of predictable and unpredictable, stories that unfold with and despite us.

Joan, I was told, was doing well. She was still on the waiting list for an apartment, but her mother was feeling better and was able to help out, so Joan had entered an outpatient drug treatment program. Timothy had been in frequently with asthma attacks, but he hadn't needed to be hospitalized again. Nobody knew exactly how Barbara and Jamal were, but Jamal had been seen a few times going to the dentist.

I asked about Teresa; nobody had seen her at the clinic. Betty had seen her once in the grocery store with Lila. "She looked awful," she said. "And she kept yelling at that poor little kid. I ducked out before she saw me."

I asked about various other families I'd wondered and worried about while I was away. Some new babies had been born into families I followed, all normal and healthy. A few children had been very sick, with things like pneumonia or asthma or high fever, but nobody had been seriously ill and all had recovered. "You are going to be so happy when you see the Molina kids," said Marta. "They are doing great." Her face lit up as she told me this. Marta really cared about the families, and would do just about anything for them. Many of the mothers had figured this out and asked specifically for her when they came to the window, in order to improve their chances of getting what they wanted.

Each time I asked about a family, Marta or Alison or whoever I was asking would have to pause and think for a while. When you are working there you concentrate on the immediate task, the family in front of you, the need to be met. Then the next task, family, or need replaces them, one after another, until the end of each exhausting day. You remember what has happened, but in your mind it is a jumble of faces and incidents, some striking, most not; they are mixed beads on a string, hard to separate.

But for each of us there are certain families who catch our eyes and our hearts, families whose beads have their own special string.

Shauna played with my hair as I made my way down the hallway, nodding hello to parents and children. It was just after Christmas, and there were still some leftover toys. Every year, Children's Hospital sent over toys to give to the children, and we usually had some other donations of new and used toys. There wasn't much left, but digging through the stuff at the bottom of the big box I found a small, slightly bedraggled but clean stuffed bear, and gave it to Shauna. She grabbed it, smiled, and gave it a kiss.

The internal waiting room was getting full and busy. One of the nurse practitioners, Sandy, was doing well child care, and was obviously overbooked. The charts of children waiting to be seen were overflowing out of the plastic box on the door and Sandy looked a little frantic, tossing her blond hair and speaking rapidly in Spanish. Children ran and played and the mothers chatted. Marta and Sarah stepped quickly and lightly around the children, bringing families into rooms and moving them out after Sandy was done. Phones were ringing in the secretaries' area, and Elisa and Betty moved about, answering phones, preparing charts, looking for a nurse when a patient was at the window, giving people messages. There was a near cacophany of voices from Pediatrics and the lobby, joining together with the motion to create a musical chaos.

It made me smile. I'd missed the chaos; I loved it. I am not an orderly person; I like some degree of mess and confusion. It feels more normal, and natural, than orderliness. And when there is chaos, there is no time or space for veneers. There is more immediacy and truth; what you see is what you get. The richness and complexity of human nature is laid out in full view.

Mostly, this is wonderful. Mostly, we get beautiful things laid out in front of us, extraordinary and ordinary. We see loving families, and sweet, innocent children; we hear stories of perseverance and compassion that are tributes to what humanity can achieve. But humanity has a dark side to its richness and complexity; veneers can serve as useful containments, and without them, all sorts of things come spilling out. We see a lot of this at the clinic: lots of anger, lots of sadness, lots of meanness, lots of desperation. People yell at us at the window, for making them wait, for not having an appointment when they want one, for not having their school physical forms ready fast enough . . . people yell at their children, swatting them, sometimes for tiny offenses . . . people yell at each other, sometimes moving to blows as we clear the waiting rooms and call Security. We see a lot of tears, and hear stories of people whose apartments have holes in the walls and are crawling with cockroaches, of people with so little money that a ten-dollar prescription is impossible, of shootings and stabbings outside the window that scare the children into recurrent nightmares and phobias, of violence within the home at the hands of boyfriends and family members, of the terrible grip of addiction—stories that stay, and haunt.

We are the products, and victims, of our circumstances. We can all have the same hearts and dreams at the beginning, but life has a way of molding us and our decisions, and small decisions can gain momentum and grow into bigger ones, like a snowball rolling down a hill. We all have the ability to rise above our circumstances and change them, although some people seem more able to do this than others—those, perhaps, who are particularly independent, creative, and determined. But even the most independent, creative, and determined need deep strength and perseverance to significantly change circumstances, and they need the unconditional support of at least one person. These can be hard to come by, and so often circumstances don't change.

The nurse practitioner who worked in Adolescent Clinic, Darla, passed through on her way back from the soda machine. She stopped to say hello to me, and welcome me back. Tall and lanky, soft-spoken, with wavy brown hair that always seemed to be falling in her face, she had a warm, genuine manner that drew people in immediately.

"I'm leaving at the end of the month," she said. "Did you hear?"

I hadn't heard, but I wasn't all that surprised. People leave a lot. A nursing assistant in Pediatrics, who had begun working a few months before I left for my leave, had left while I was gone, as had one of the nutritionists and a front-desk secretary.

"I just can't take it anymore," said Darla. "I get to know these kids, and care about them, and then they're in gangs, or they're dropping out of school, or they're pregnant, or they get HIV—it's just too hard."

Her voice was tired, and she was thinner than I remembered her. She pushed her hair away from her face, and sighed. "So I got a job at a women's clinic in the suburbs, doing gyn exams. It's just part-time, too. It's going to be a little tough financially, but I can't do full-time right now. I need to rest and do some healing."

To make a difference, you need to really care. But when you really care it can hurt too much, and then you leave. I would have to be careful, I thought, although I didn't know how.

As I thought that, I realized just how very much I wanted to stay at Martha Eliot. Yes, the practice of medicine was more complicated and more frustrating there. Yes, the world of the inner city was different from anything I'd known before and was sometimes a difficult place to be. But I felt useful there, felt like I had more to contribute there than anywhere else. And I liked the people so very much.

Darla said good-bye and went upstairs. I sat down in an empty chair with Shauna on my lap, and as she played with the bear I watched the children around me. A curly-haired toddler in a pink jumpsuit clung to her mother's leg, hiding behind it when I looked at her and then peering around to stare at Shauna's bear. Another toddler, who had just gotten a shot, huddled in his mother's lap. He buried his tear-stained face in her breasts as he tried to stop crying; she kissed his head and stroked his dark hair. An older girl, maybe nine or ten, bounced an infant on her knee carefully and confidently, keeping an eye on two little boys who were playing on the floor in front of her. They began to fight over a toy car; quickly, the girl swooped down, and with a few quick, stern words in Spanish she took the car from one, gave it to the other, and handed the first another toy car from the big diaper bag at her feet. The boys hesitated a moment, and then went back to playing, happily rolling the cars toward each other. The toddler in the pink jumpsuit wandered over on tiptoes to watch them, wide-eyed, as if hypnotized by the toy cars going back and forth. The other toddler stopped crying; he watched the cars too and smiled.

Working with children is easier than working with adolescents or adults. The children are still so full of potential, blank slates on which maybe wonderful things will be written; there is still much reason for hope.

Shauna started to fuss, apparently bored with the bear, so I brought her back to the exam room where her mother and brother were. Her brother was sitting alone on the table, smiling, breathing more comfortably. His mother sat in the chair, and when she saw Shauna she smiled and reached for her. Shauna grinned and threw herself toward her mother, as if she thought she could fly to her; I guided her into her mother's arms.

The pile of charts of children waiting to be seen had grown; I grabbed one off the top. I didn't want to do follow-up or read my mail anymore. Suddenly, I wanted to get to work.

"I was dreaming that . . . that I was president!" Charlie said, holding his arms up in a grand gesture. He was explaining to me why he wet the bed. "Yeah, I was dreaming that I was president and I just didn't wake up."

"Every night you dream that you're the president?" I asked.

"No," he said with a mischevious smile. "Some nights I dream that I'm an astronaut."

He was six years old, wiry, in constant motion even when sitting down. He seemed very eager to please; his eyes frequently tried to catch mine and whenever they did, he smiled at me.

His new foster mother had brought him to the clinic because of bed-wetting. She was his third foster mother; he came to live with her a month before so that he would be with his brother, a brother he had never met. The baby was nine months old, born long after Charlie was taken away from his mother. She used drugs and wouldn't stop.

His new foster mother, Señora Ortega, spoke Spanish. Her English was an assorted vocabulary of mispronounced words and grammatically incorrect sentences. She and Charlie seemed to understand one another, though. He was learning some Spanish, as I discovered when I asked Señora Ortega a question in Spanish and Charlie answered me.

"It's not every night," he said indignantly. "I only wet the bed sometimes."

I talked about using positive reinforcement to decrease the bed-wetting, about rewarding Charlie for staying dry rather than punishing him for wetting. Señora Ortega wasn't really listening to me. She would do it her own way, I knew. She had a house full of foster children and so was in the clinic often; I had come to know her well. She would do something like hang his wet pajamas up where everyone could see, to humiliate him out of his habit. I wondered why she bothered to bring him to the clinic.

I went and got one of the leftover Christmas toys for Charlie: a little plastic plane with a parachute that could be attached to it. The parachute had lots of thin strings, and as Charlie ripped open the package, the strings got tangled. He worked at untangling them for a while, but somehow he just tangled them more.

"Can I help?" I said.

He looked up at me, stared at me. It was as if he was surprised, as if someone helping would never have occurred to him. He hesitated.

"No, I can do it," he said.

He worked the strings out more or less straight, tied them to the airplane in not quite the right place, and threw it into the air. It flew briefly, crookedly, and then crashed to the floor; the parachute only partially opened. I started to say something, like an apology, but then I saw Charlie's face. He was grinning.

"That's cool," he said.

It was free, he did it himself, and it sort of worked. What more could this little boy ask for? I looked at his bright, hopeful face and I was full of angry sadness.

Without even thinking, I was down on the floor, picking up the plane, dusting it off and untangling the strings. I wanted to make it soar for him.

Twelve

It took a long time for Teresa to get into the exam room.

Lila ran in ahead of me, dragging her coat along the floor, and spun around to show me her dress; it was a birthday present from her aunt, she told me. It was pink and frilly, and had what looked like a few days' worth of food stains and wrinkles.

Damian limped in, but even still he was faster than Teresa. He had obviously hurt his knee—his jeans were torn there and stained with some dried blood—but he wouldn't answer any of my questions about it. He sat down in one of the chairs, huddled in the winter coat that was much too big for him, and stared at the floor.

Teresa came in as if dragging her legs with her. She wore a stretched-out cotton sweater over a dirty denim skirt, and a gray wool overcoat with a couple of holes in it. She sat down slowly and unsteadily in the other chair. I stayed standing, leaning against the exam table, because there was nowhere else to sit and I wasn't about to ask either of them to give up a chair.

"Are you okay?" I asked Teresa.

"Ain't nothing wrong with me," she said gruffly. "We's here for Lila's appointment, and I asked the nurse could I bring Damian in 'cause he gone and hurt himself again."

"What happened?"

Damian was still staring at the floor.

"Tell the doctor what happened," said Teresa.

He was silent and motionless in the chair.

"Would you tell the doctor what fuckin' happened! What's your problem!" Her voice was so loud and shrill it startled me. It didn't seem to startle Damian or Lila.

Damian shrugged. "I just fell," he said softly.

"The fuck you just fell," said Teresa, her voice still shrill. "You and your friends was running away from them cops." She turned to me. "That's what his father's neighbors told me, and I knows they's telling the truth. They didn't know why the cops was chasing them, though, and he won't tell me nothin'."

I reached under the exam table and got out a gown. "Put this on over your clothes," I said to Damian, "and then take off your pants." He scowled, but stood up slowly and took the gown from me. He took off his coat, put the gown on over his sweatshirt, and slid off the jeans.

"He's gettin' to be trouble, this kid," said Teresa. "He don't listen to nobody. His father, he 'bout had it with him, so he lets him do what he want so's he's out of his hair."

I motioned Damian up onto the exam table and looked at his knee. He had a large abrasion, but it wasn't serious and didn't need stitches. I washed it and put on some ointment and a bandage. Damian didn't look at me at all.

I looked through his chart. "He needs a physical," I said. "It has been almost three years."

"Tell his father," said Teresa. "I ain't got custody of him."

Her head was in her hands; she looked up at me with bloodshot eyes.

"Look, I try makin' appointments for him but it don't work out 'cause his father don't cooperate and these days, Damian don't neither. We ain't got no regular visitation thing no more—his father drops him off when he feels like it and when he can catch him. I only know 'bout his knee 'cause I was over here with Lila and the neighbors stopped me." Her voice was heavy with exhaustion.

"I'll call his father," I said.

Damian's pants were back on within seconds and he was back in his coat and the chair. Lila climbed up on the table and grinned at me. "My turn!" she said triumphantly. She looked exactly the same as she had the last time I saw her, except that she had blue beads in her hair instead of white ones.

The blood tests from Lila's physical had shown that she was anemic, and I had prescribed some iron. I'd made an appointment for her a couple of months after that to check her weight and see if her anemia was improving, but she didn't show. I tried to call Teresa, and Lila's father, but both phones were disconnected. Before I went on maternity leave, I sent a letter to the address listed for Lila in the computer, which was her father's address. I was hoping she would come in while I was gone. She hadn't. It was now more than six months since the physical.

"How long did Lila take the iron?" I asked.

"I dunno," said Teresa. "I went and got it from the pharmacy and I gave it to her father. I don't know how long he gave it. Probably not long, knowin' him."

"What about when she was with you?"

"He kept forgettin' to bring it with her, and finally I stopped askin' 'bout it." Her voice was getting harder to hear, and more slurred.

"Okay," I said slowly. It wasn't okay, of course, but it didn't feel worthwhile to argue with her right then. "Well, we'll check her blood today and see what we need to do. Lila, hop down and let's weigh you."

Lila jumped off into my arms, giving me a hug as she did so. I brought her to the scale and helped her take off her shoes. She hadn't gained any weight since her physical.

"She don't eat," said Teresa softly. She was slumped in the chair.

"Guys, why don't you wait outside in the waiting room here," I said to the children. "There are some toys and some crayons and paper. I want to talk to your mother." They left quickly, obviously happy to go.

"Damian ain't gonna be there, watch," said Teresa. "He's gonna leave."

I shut the door. I brought the chair Damian had been sitting in closer to Teresa, and sat down.

"Please tell me what's going on," I said. "I'm worried about you."

"I'm okay."

"You're not okay. You look terrible, you clearly don't feel well. What's wrong? Are you sick?"

"I ain't sick," she said.

I paused for a second. "Are you using?" I asked tentatively.

"I'm not using," she snapped. "I been clean."

"That's great," I said, a little too enthusiastically. "So . . . ?"

"I'm pregnant, okay?" she said. "I'm pregnant and I feel like shit and I feel like getting high but I'm not. Sorry if I don't look so pretty."

I sat back in the chair. We were both silent.

"I'm sorry for thinking you were using," I said. "Is there anything I can do? Is there anything you need?"

Teresa laughed; it was more of a sigh than a laugh. "Anything I need? Sure, I needs lots of things. Like a different life. You can get me that?"

I shifted in the chair, opened my mouth, and closed it again.

Teresa leaned forward again, her elbows on her knees. "Yeah, a different life, I ain't never gonna get that. This baby, though, I want him to be okay, so I's gonna keep clean this time. The other times, I'd slip a little. This time, I ain't gonna slip. I'd like to keep this baby, and if I slip, they's always finding out and takin' my babies."

"Who's the father?" I asked.

"Lila's daddy," she said. "We been gettin' along okay, he comes by to see me. Ronald's daddy, he came over once recently trying to see me, but I wouldn't let him in. Started bangin' on the door, he did, but I don't let him in. He used to beat me, did you know that? Is it in some chart somewhere?" Her voice rose.

"I didn't know that," I said.

"What do you got in those charts of yours, anyway? You folks who stare at me like I'm some piece of shit—you got the truth about my life? I dropped out of school when I was fourteen, and I swear, nobody noticed. I never understood that. Don't the school call or somethin'? How did they not notice? Nobody in my family paid no attention to me 'less they wanted somethin' from me. Friends of my parents, they had me sellin' marijuana for them, nobody noticed that neither."

Her bloodshot eyes looked like they were on fire, and she sat up straight.

"I wanted to be a singer. Everybody always said I should be a singer. I'd sneak into clubs with my cousin, and I'd sing, and the people, they'd clap and clap for me. I was doing the drugs a little then—not much, just some so I could hang out with them people and they'd take me with them to clubs and stuff and I'd sing. Everybody always said I should make a record. But then I started havin' the babies, and the drugs got worse, and here I am."

She had me, and she knew it. Her fiery eyes sparkled a little and her hand went up, like a lecturer emphasizing the important points.

"I's lucky I didn't have babies 'fore I did," she said. "I didn't know what I was doin'. My mother's friend, she told me I had to be nice to men when they was nice to me. She was real clear what she meant, and I believed her. I was too young to know any better. I was stoned out of my mind most the time, no idea what I was doing. I was constantly seein' people gettin' high, and they was so content. I wanted to be content like that."

She spoke quickly, the words stumbling over each other sometimes as if they couldn't get out fast enough. She was talking to me but really it felt like she was talking to the room, or the air, talking just so that the words were said.

"Kept clean just about all the pregnancy with Damian. I didn't want to hurt my baby. Slipped a couple of times, but I wasn't with DSS then, they weren't watching me. He came out fine, I was real happy with him. I was going to make a nice life for us, me and my baby. But I couldn't get no job, seeing's as how I had trouble filling out them applications, for all the good school did me, and didn't have no skills, so I's stuck on welfare and nobody to watch my baby to go to no school and all my friends, they use. There weren't nothin' else to do finally but use and I hated myself but that's what I ended up doin'."

"How could you take care of children while you were using?"

"It ain't so hard. People do it all the time, you folks just don't understand. I'd get 'em all fed first, get 'em their toys so they don't bother me none or be needin' anything, change 'em, whatever. I'd lock the apartment door so's the kids couldn't go wanderin' and then I'd go in the bathroom and shut the door tight so they didn't see me. I never let 'em see me takin' the stuff. I don't want 'em followin' my example, you know. And I was never so stoned that my kids wasn't clean or fed. My kids was always clean and fed."

"Who reported you to DSS?"

"Ronald's father. He was mad at me 'cause I called the police on him. He gave me a big old black eye. He said he'd get back at me 'cause he had to spend the night in jail. Called up DSS as soon as he got out. They came and took the babies and they been on me ever since. I keep thinkin' maybe I'm gonna stay clean but it just don't happen."

Her hand, which had stayed in the air, came down slowly, and fell into her lap. Teresa stared at it, as if it were something unfamiliar. She turned it over and looked at her palm before slowly drawing her hand into a fist.

"What could make it happen?" I asked hesitantly.

The fire had gone out in the bloodshot eyes that looked dully past me. "I don't know," she said slowly. "I wake up in the morning and it's all so dirty and there's nothin' there. I want to keep clean for this baby so he's born okay and I don't hurt him. But I can't think any further than that. I can't make no plans."

I reached out to touch her arm but she moved, slightly but definitively, out of reach. She reached behind her head and tightened her bandanna, then leaned back in the chair, stretched out her legs, and looked me in the eye.

"I'll try to get Lila to eat some more," she said firmly. "Where's the form for the blood test?"

I handed it to her. She stood up and walked to the door.

"I want to help you," I said.

"I know you do," she said. "But you can't."

Thirteen

I started to read the newspaper differently.

Before I worked at Martha Eliot, I would read the front section of *The Boston Globe* and the Op-Eds first, then flip through the Living/Arts section, maybe glance at the front page of Metro/Region if I had time. But when I started to get to know the patients at Martha Eliot I began to glance at the headlines in the front section, then go straight to the Metro/Region section, where I would carefully look at each story. I was worried about events and decisions that might affect my patients. I checked each of the small stories about shootings and stabbings and robberies, looking for familiar names and streets. I wanted to be sure nothing bad had happened to anyone I knew.

Most of the people involved in the shootings and stabbings and robberies were young men, and I usually wasn't sure if I knew them or not. With some notable exceptions, the fathers and the older brothers and cousins were largely shadowy figures to me. Sometimes I would meet a father briefly; he usually sat silently in a chair in the room or waited in the waiting room, talking me with me only if pressed to do so, and then uncomfortably. So many of the fathers were living separately from the family, marginally and intermittently involved. I read the newspaper and I hoped that the young man who was killed not too far from the clinic and had the same last name as a family I knew wasn't the father in that family, or a brother or a cousin.

But even if he wasn't, he was probably somebody's father, or brother, or cousin. And he was certainly somebody's son.

I was raised in wealthy, tranquil suburbia, where I learned to be suspicious of any young man I saw in the inner city, where I came to think of the people who perpetrated violent crime as "bad guys" who needed punishment and then rehabilitation. But now, after walking through the housing development and along the streets of the communities my patients called home, after getting to know so many families and visiting the schools, this view was becoming less and less workable. I was beginning to see crime as a way of making a way in the world, as a way of getting by and making money—not a legal or safe way, but a way nonetheless.

I watched Joan's son Jamal, and Teresa's son Damian, and the other boys I saw at the clinic. In the exam room, dressed in a hospital gown with their mother sitting in the chair nearby, they acted more or less like any other boy their age, although perhaps a little more sullen. But when the gowns came off and the clothes went back on and they were back out in the waiting room they were different. Their speech took on the jargon of the street, their steps had a swagger, their shoulders hunched slightly forward, and their eyes took on a dull watchfulness. They became caricatures of the young men of the inner-city streets. Soon, I feared, they could move from being caricatures to being apprentices.

Any child, every child, watches the world around him and picks his dreams, thinks about what he wants to be when he grows up. He picks out people to be heroes, people he wants to be like. These people can be anybody—but there is usually something about their lives that the child wants to have. Maybe the person seems very happy, or helps people, or has an exciting job, or just seems to enjoy life. Often the person will have some power that the child sees as positive, and will have the respect of others in the community. Often the person will have money, enough to buy things that the child sees as the kinds of toys he wants to have when he grows up.

When I ask the little children what they want to be when they grow up they talk about Superman and Batman and other superheroes they watch on television, or they say teacher or fireman, or the other simple things they learn about in the early years of school. Interestingly, the children I see at Martha Eliot rarely say they want to be policemen, probably because distrust of policemen is so common there. Sometimes they say they want to be a doctor, smiling at me.

The older children are less quick to answer; they have begun to be realistic, and they have begun to look around them for role models. We hope that the child picks his hardworking father or uncle, or his minister or doctor, or his mother steadfastly pursuing her education—and follows in one of their footsteps. But I know from the very long time some children take to answer, from the completely blank looks and shrugs that they frequently give me, that some families don't have many such role models to offer.

In the inner city there can be other prominent people in the child's world, people he may see every day on the street corners or in the expensive cars, people he certainly hears about if he doesn't see them: the gangs and the drug dealers. They have much for the child to envy: friends, power, the respect of others (or their fear, but the child may only see that as respect), money. Their lives may seem much more glamorous, exciting, and lucrative than the lives of the hardworking people he knows, and professions like medicine or law may seem impossible to attain because of all the schooling involved. There are professional people who bring their children to the clinic, people who have college degrees and sometimes even some more—but they are relatively few. Many of the children I see at Martha Eliot have nobody in their family who has finished college. Some of them have nobody in the family who has finished high school.

It's all about options, or at least about perceived options, which are the only real ones. The child of the inner city may see gangs and dealing drugs as the most reliable way for him to make money and his way in the world. He may see being part of a gang as the best way to have friends who really care about him—and the best way to keep himself protected on the street. He may come to see violence as the only effective way to solve disputes, because that is the only effective way he has seen.

I read the stories in the newspaper, the brief little ones about the deaths and violent crimes, and I found myself wondering about the people involved—these people who could be the father, or brother, or child of someone I know. How did he come to be slouched in that car with that gun in his hand when that bullet exploded through his brain? Why was this the option he chose? When he was little did he dream of anything else? Did he like the life he led? If not, did he see a way out—or was he just waiting to die? Or, if he was very young, did he not quite realize that death was possible?

Then I read the stories about the governor's and the mayor's and the candidate's plans to reduce crime. More police on the street, they would say. Stricter gun control. Mandatory jail sentences, and long ones. And while I thought that these things would help, the stories seemed remote and disconnected from the stories about the crimes themselves, or from the people who were becoming so very real to me—and they seemed to miss the point.

There were frequently stories in the newspaper about welfare and "welfare reform," which I always read carefully. The basic premise seemed to be that too many people were living comfortably off the government instead of getting their act together and getting jobs. Before I started working at Martha Eliot, this made sense to me, not that I thought about it very much. But within a few months of working with family after family on welfare, it began to seem less straightforward.

First of all, it is not a comfortable life. The welfare check is not a lot of money. It pays for food, because food stamps and WIC, the government program for pregnant and nursing women and young children, rarely cover the monthly food bill. It pays for clothes and diapers, as long as they are cheap. It pays the rent—but only if the rent is subsidized. Without a subsidy, rent here in the Boston area would likely eat up the whole welfare check, so those who are unable to get a subsidy must find a place to share, or at least someone to stay with for a while. It pays, one hopes, for utilities—but there may or may not be enough left for the phone bill, and many of our families don't have phones. Everything becomes a trade-off: if you buy your child a toy, there may not be enough for underwear; if you buy cough medicine, you may be short on the rent.

Life on welfare is a day to day, subsistence existence, and an existence kept firmly within poverty. There isn't much that's attractive about it. You don't have to work, that's true. But essentially everyone I know who is on welfare has children, and they aren't exactly living lives of leisure as they try to keep up with the demands of raising children and keeping a home, tasks that are more difficult to do when you are poor.

Not that everyone on welfare knew it would be like that ahead of time. I remember one mother on welfare laughing and saying to me, "I sit here and listen to these kids, young kids, pregnant, thinking it's a big thing to have a baby and be on welfare. I was the same way when I grew up: 'Shoot, you don't have to do nothing, they just pay you for staying in the house and everything,' I said. Then I went on welfare." She went on welfare and the money was gone to feed and clothe the children as soon as it came in and when she tried to supplement it with part-time work her check was cut . . . it wasn't at all what she thought it would be.

I've asked many women if when they were younger they had expected that they would end up on welfare. Most of them say no. They thought they'd have jobs, or be married to men who would support them and their children. One woman who grew up on welfare said, "I used to be embarrassed that my mother was on welfare. You see the other kids in school with nice clothes, who have money, who go to school with food. I used to say to myself that I would never be on welfare when I grew up." But then she fell in love and got pregnant. Her boyfriend left her, and the part-time job she had as a chambermaid didn't offer insurance let alone cover expenses . . . so she quit and went on welfare. It was only temporary, she told herself, but temporary had extended itself into five years.

Lots of the mothers I see at the clinic tell similar stories, of dreams that were derailed. Often it is pregnancy that does the derailing. The women talk about getting pregnant by accident, or because they were in love, or because they wanted a baby to love. But babies have a way of narrowing choices, because of all the time and money they require. Sometimes it is being left to care alone for children that does the derailing; mothers tell stories of trying to no avail to get child support from the fathers of their children, and of being unable to support the family on their salaries alone.

Some of the women, when asked if they expected to be on welfare, frown and shrug and say that they *did* sort of expect it. It was what they saw everyone doing when they were growing up. They got pregnant because their friends did and they didn't have any-thing else they particularly wanted to do with their lives, and they went on welfare because their friends did and they didn't really know what else to do. It wasn't a life they really liked, but they didn't see any other real option.

There are other options, of course. For instance, teenage moth-ers could stay with their parents rather than using welfare to go out on their own—provided those parents are willing and capable, which many of them are not. And certainly, obviously, the women could get a job. Some people are indeed lazy; some people do fit the stereotype, and are milking the system for all it's worth. But I have run into very few such people. Most people I've met would rather be off welfare than on it.

I'm sure that there are educated women on welfare, but the vast majority of women on welfare that I see at Martha Eliot have just a high school diploma, if that, with few marketable skills. Let's face it, the job possibilities open to them are limited. The ones I know who have found jobs do things like factory assembly or office cleaning. They work as store cashiers or in fast-food restaurants or in laundries or do part-time jobs for which they are paid under the table. None of these jobs pay very much money, and few offer health insurance, especially affordable family plans to cover the children too. Families moving off welfare have a grace period of sorts during which they can keep their Medicaid benefits and get a day care subsidy, but once that time is over families are left on their own to achieve what may very well be impossible.

Somehow, an appreciation of these realities is markedly missing from the political rhetoric about welfare reform, and this is why the use of the words "welfare reform" seems ridiculous to me. The way it is currently formulated isn't about "reform," unless you want to define reform as simply spending less money. And the human cost of this "reform" is going to be huge, especially for children born innocently into families on or considering welfare. Far too many of them will go hungry and have no place to live. Far too many of them won't have ready access to health care and will be sick, or sicker, or even die because of this. Unfortunately, it looks like these policy decisions have been made, over the protests of those of us who actually deal with these families face-to-face, day after day. There is not much to do now but scramble to find whatever help we can for people and hope that not too many children starve, freeze, or die of preventable or treatable illnesses before those in positions of power realize that this particular kind of reform was a bad idea.

Fourteen

The woman holding the baby huddled over him, surrounding him with herself as if he were still inside her. Her long black hair was pulled back tightly away from her face and rolled into a bun held neatly with bobby pins against the back of her head. The brown sweater she wore clung tightly, too, defining her small, delicate arms and torso. Her skin was the color of milk chocolate, and when she looked up at me her eyes, carefully outlined in blue eyeliner, were so dark they were almost black.

She did not look up at me for long, just enough to be polite as she answered my questions in Spanish—and then her eyes were quickly down, back to the half-asleep baby in her lap who whimpered softly, uncomfortably, with his fever. He had her chocolate-colored skin and black hair and her delicateness; he was thin and small for four months.

The baby, Kevin, had sickle-cell anemia. His red blood cells were made wrong, and sometimes twisted and clumped in his arteries and veins, blocking the flow of blood. This could cause him pain, and damage to his body, and make it hard for him to fight infection when his blood, full of its weapons against infection, couldn't get where it needed to go. And there were never enough of the red cells; he would always be anemic, always at risk of tiring easily, always making his heart work harder.

Sickle-cell anemia is something you are born with, a piece of genetic bad luck. Both of Kevin's parents were carriers, meaning that they each had one copy of the sickle-cell gene. Having one copy can be a good thing: it doesn't cause significant health problems, and when some of your red cells are made differently, it helps protect you from malaria. And when two carriers have a child together, the odds are only one in four that the child will get two copies of the gene. But when you have two copies of the gene, when all of your red cells are made differently, it is a terrible disease.

There was a man in the room, too. Tall, thin, and unshaven, he stood against the wall in the corner, watching the woman and me. He had not spoken since I entered the room; when I introduced myself he just nodded. He did not tell me his name; the woman told me that his name was Ricardo, and that he was Kevin's father. The woman's name was Luz, which means "light" in Spanish.

I asked if I could examine the baby; reluctantly, Luz lifted him from her lap and gave him to me. I brought him to the exam table and laid him down; his eyes stayed closed. He was breathing quickly and his skin was hot with fever. His heart was beating rapidly and there was a murmur, most probably from the fever and the anemia. I could feel his spleen, made large from trying to catch and clear away the clumped red blood cells. His ears and throat looked fine. It could be a virus causing his fever, or it could be bacteria, or something else. He would need more tests to find out. But most important, he needed to be admitted to the hospital for observation and antibiotics. Because of his disease, every illness could possibly be life-threatening.

He opened his eyes and looked up at me. His eyes were brown, not dark brown like Luz's but instead a warm, melting brown, and so big I felt like I could fall inside them. It took my breath away; they were the exact same eyes as my son's. Kevin had Zachary's eyes.

I could feel Ricardo staring at me; I turned and he was frowning, leaning forward slightly, watching my every move. He clearly did not trust me.

"El es muy lindo," I said to him—he's very handsome—hoping that it might help. There was a flicker of something across his eyes, perhaps pride, but the frown remained. Luz smiled broadly.

She, too, leaned forward, but it was a different sort of leaning forward. She trusted me, but she wanted Kevin back.

I picked him up and handed him back; her thin arms came reaching out as soon as I moved toward her, gathering him in close to her body again. She ran her fingertips along his cheek; he smiled at her.

Ricardo's eyes were on Luz now, moving over every inch of her, hawklike, as if memorizing. He moved closer to her and the baby, although he still stood away, near the wall. His black pants and white shirt were clean and pressed, contrasting oddly with his unkempt dark hair and unshaven face. He wore a leather jacket that looked new.

I explained why Kevin needed to go over to the hospital to be admitted. Luz's eyes filled with tears, but she nodded. She had been told, when Kevin was first diagnosed with sickle-cell disease, that he would be admitted whenever he had a fever.

"*¿Puedo quedar con él?*" she asked—can I stay with him?

"*Claro,*" I said—of course. "*Y su padre también, si quiere,*" I said, motioning to Ricardo—and he can too, if he wants.

Luz's dark eyes narrowed slightly and her shoulders stiffened. She glanced quickly at Ricardo, although she did not meet his intense gaze.

"*Ricardo tiene que trabajar,*" she said—he has to go to work.

Ricardo looked at me, directly but blankly.

"*Voy a ir con ellos,*" he said. "*Me quedaré lo más que pueda.*" His voice was deep, gravelly, and a little stern. He would go with them, and stay as long as he could. He put his hand on Luz's back. She smiled at him, but it looked a little forced.

I went to the hospital to see them at around seven the next morning. The shade was down in Kevin's room; as my eyes adjusted to the dark, I saw that his crib was empty. He was on the cot that was next to the crib, with Luz. They were both asleep. Luz lay tangled in the white hospital sheets, wearing the same clothes she'd been wearing the day before at the clinic; Kevin lay on his side, his hands and feet touching her arm, his face close enough to hers to feel her breath. An IV giving him fluids and antibiotics went into his left arm, which was held out straight against a cloth-covered board, fastened with lots of white tape.

I sat down on the edge of the cot and touched Luz's shoulder to wake her. Her eyes flew open and she sat up quickly, waking Kevin as she did. When she saw it was me she sighed and her shoulders relaxed.

"Lo siento," I said, apologizing for waking her.

"No, está bien," she said—it's okay. She smiled at me and scooped up Kevin, who had started to whimper. Once in her arms he fell back to sleep.

I asked how the night had been; she shrugged and said that it was long and they were woken up a lot by the nurses checking on Kevin, but his fever was down.

I pulled my stethoscope out of my bag and listened to his chest. His heart was beating less rapidly than it had been the day before. With him still in her arms, I ran my hands over him, looking for anything new or different from the day before: enlarged lymph nodes, any change in his liver or spleen, any swelling of his hands or feet, which can happen when the blood vessels are blocked. I found nothing.

He was better, I told Luz, but he needed to stay for at least another day for observation and to be sure that the blood tests didn't show any bacteria. She nodded. I asked her what she thought of the hospital; her eyes lit up and she said that she had never seen anything like it before.

I laughed. *"¿De donde es Ud.?"* I asked—where are you from?

She was from a village in the Dominican Republic, she told me, a very small village where things were very different. It was very poor, which was why she left—there was much more here, and now with Kevin's illness she didn't think she could ever go back. She wanted him to have the very best, and there were no hospitals like this one anywhere near her village. But it was beautiful there, and her mother was there, and she missed it because it was home.

Her Spanish was simple, but she was very articulate and expressive. Her face lit up as she spoke, keeping her voice down so as not to wake the baby. Her hair was loose and tangled, and the blue eyeliner was smudged, but there was something about the way she carried herself that made her elegant.

"*¿Donde está Ricardo?*" I asked. A shadow passed over her face. She didn't know where he was, she said. He was probably working.

I asked if he lived with her; she said no, she had her own place. He lived with his family. She clearly didn't want to talk about him.

I asked, awkwardly, if everything was okay between her and Ricardo. She shrugged. She said that he helped out, giving her rides to the doctor and to the store, and money to buy things for the baby. And then she abruptly changed the subject, asking if Kevin was going to need any more tests.

"*Una prueba de sangre esta mañana,*" I said—one blood test this morning.

"*Ay, pobrecito, no es justo,*" she said—poor baby, it's not fair.

She looked up at me and asked if I could hold him a moment while she went to the bathroom. Of course, I said, and held out my arms for his small, soft body. Her eyes were red; she ducked quickly into the adjoining bathroom, shutting the door softly.

I looked down at him sleeping against me, at the rise and fall of his chest and his smooth, perfect skin, and thought, She's right. It's not fair. He did nothing to deserve this illness, this terrible illness that was going to make his life shorter and very painful. And there was nothing that could have prevented it, either. It was a matter of chance: the chance that Luz and Ricardo met, the chance that the genes fell together the way they did. It was one of those accidents of birth. So many powerful things are decided for us in that moment of conception: our parents, our genes, the situation into which we are born. These things make and change our lives forever, and we cannot control them.

He was just so like Zachary. He was the same age, he had the same eyes, and he filled my arms just the same way. Tears came to my eyes as I thought about what might have been for my child, and what might still be: who knew, really, what the falling together of Mark's and my genes had caused, what the chance of our meeting would mean for our children.

Luz came out of the bathroom and took Kevin from me, slipping one dark, slender hand under his head and the other under the small of his back, lifting him and bringing him to her body as she sat down beside me on the cot.

"*¿No hay tratamiento para él?*" she asked—was there no treatment for him?

I was confused. I said that there were treatments for infections and fever.

She shook her head. "*Para su falcemia,*" she said.

I paused, and swallowed. There were treatments to help him feel better, I told her, but there was nothing that would cure sickle-cell disease. Maybe there would be in the future, but there was nothing now.

She looked down at Kevin and her eyes got red again.

I didn't know what to say. They don't teach you what to say in this situation while you're in medical school. They don't teach you much in general about what to say to patients and families, but this particular area is especially difficult for physicians. Medical training is oriented around problem solving, around fixing and curing. That is how we see our job; that is how we help people. It is the image we enter medical school with: the shining doctor in the white coat who swoops in with the solution and some words of wisdom as well. It is an image that persists and is encouraged during our training; it has tremendous appeal in its simplicity and power.

We just try to do the same thing when faced with unsolvable problems. We try to swoop in with the solution and the wisdom— and finding ourselves lacking in both, we mutter often useless things and scurry off, hoping that the next patient's problems can be solved.

"*¿Hay algo que puedo hacer?*" I asked—is there anything I can do?

She looked up at me with her dark, reddened eyes, smiled half-heartedly, and shook her head.

I asked her to call if she needed me. I said that I would be back the next day, but I could come back sooner if anything happened or if she needed me. I didn't know what she would need me for, but it was all I could think of to say. I picked up my coat and my back-pack, said good-bye, and left.

Fifteen

B ickford Street stops abruptly in front of the old clinic. On some maps it looks like it goes all the way through to Centre Street but actually there is a section, maybe five yards long, where there is something of a pedestrian area and cars can't get through. So when the snowplows come in the winter to clear Bickford Street, all the snow is dumped from either side onto the pedestrian area and it makes a pile several feet high. During particularly snowy winters, like the one after I had Zack, the pile becomes a hill. And the hill, of course, fills with children.

One day in late February I came in around one; I had a dentist appointment, so I had taken the morning off. Usually I came in early and left late, so I didn't get to see the children playing outside. It was school vacation week, and there were about a dozen children playing on the pile. Most were dressed very warmly, with not just winter coats and hats but snowpants and waterproof mittens, but some wore lightweight jackets and no mittens or hat. None of them looked cold, though. They were laughing and yelling, struggling to climb the icy sides to the top and then sliding, tumbling, down to the bottom on top of each other.

A young girl, wearing a dirty blue winter coat and a pair of women's gloves that were too big for her, walked along the bottom of the pile, watching the others go down, catching the smaller ones as they approached the pavement. She walked along like a sentinel, her hands behind her back when they weren't catching snowsuited, squirmy children. As I stopped in front of the pile to watch, she looked over at me, and I realized that I knew her. It was Joan's daughter.

"Barbara," I said. "How are you?"

She smiled and came over to me. "I'm fine," she said. "I'm just watching the kids. They don't watch where they're going real well."

"I saw you," I said. "You're nice to look out for them."

She smiled shyly and pushed back her braids. "Someone's gotta make sure they don't get hurt," she said.

"How's your mother?" I asked.

She seemed to hesitate, although I wasn't entirely sure. "She's fine," she said, looking away. "She's coming over in a few minutes to see you with the baby—he's wheezing again."

"Oh, that's too bad. He has been wheezing a lot, hasn't he?"

"Yeah," said Barbara, staring at the snowpile. Then she turned to me. "It's not my mother's fault. She always gives him the medicine." Her eyes looked intently into mine.

"Of course it's not her fault," I said, surprised.

"She always calls and brings him over when he starts up with the wheezing, too," continued Barbara, still grabbing my eyes with hers. "She always does what she 'sposed to."

"Yes, she does," I said, feeling almost hypnotized by her dark eyes. "Barbara, is something going on?"

She turned away, and put her hands behind her back again. "Nothing. We're doing great."

"If there is something going on, maybe I could help."

She turned back to me, and frowned slightly. "We're doing great," she said again. "My mother, though, she been real busy. There's all the shopping and the cleaning and laundry and stuff, and Jamal and me, we's always needing help with our homework, so she don't get much time free to go to them NA meetings."

"It must be hard for her," I said as a snowball whizzed past my ear toward the snowpile, hitting a little boy, who started to cry.

I turned and looked behind me. A group of boys were pointing at the pile and laughing. There were six of them, of different ages and sizes, none older than about thirteen.

"Jamal Johnson!" said Barbara loudly and sternly. "Jamal Johnson, I saw you throw that snowball. Get over here."

The boys stopped laughing, and Jamal emerged from the center of the group. He wore a ripped red jacket and red mittens with holes, and a black wool hat with the Boston Bruins insignia was pulled down over his ears. He sauntered over, a mixture of cocky and contrite.

"So I threw it, so what?" he said, deepening his voice and putting his hands on his hips. He did not look at Barbara, though; he looked past her, at the brick of the building behind her.

"What do you mean, so what?" said Barbara, moving closer to him so that she was talking right into his face. He tried to back away but she moved closer again. "You hit that little kid over there and made him cry, and you nearly hit the doctor."

He looked up at me and took his hands off his hips.

"Now, you say you're sorry, Jamal Johnson," said Barbara, more softly but just as sternly.

He looked at me and at the little boy, who had stopped crying and was sitting uninjured at the bottom of the snowpile watching Barbara and Jamal. He looked behind him. The group of boys had run off to join four older boys who were leaning against the wall behind the Dumpster, and were no longer paying any attention to him.

"Sorry," he said quickly, and ran to join the boys.

I turned to talk to Barbara, but she had run to the snowpile to catch a little girl careening down backward.

Inside it was quiet, as it was still lunchtime. I followed the trail of muddy footprints into Pediatrics and found the last spare hanger in the coat closet, which also served as a storage space for cans of formula.

The staff room was empty. I pulled my mail out of the mailbox and checked my messages, which were stuck with Scotch tape to "my" section of the shelf on the wall. There was a message from Tom Henry, Joan's DSS worker, asking me to call him. I sat down on one of the bright orange chairs, picked up the phone, and called him immediately.

"Thanks for calling back," he said. "I just wanted to touch base with you. I'm kind of worried about Joan."

"Why?"

"You know, it's nothing real specific. I made a couple of appointments to meet her to go to the Housing office with her, and she didn't show. And a couple of times I've gone by her mother's apartment to visit, appointments I set up with her, and she's not there. Her mother's always got some reason, like that she needed to take Timothy to the clinic or she needed to run out to the store."

"I personally haven't seen that much of her. I was on maternity leave, and I work part-time," I said. "But I know that she *has* been in here a lot with Timothy. His asthma has been bad this winter."

"Maybe that's all it is with the appointments. I hope so. She tells me that she goes to Narcotics Anonymous meetings, but she never has the signature I ask for from the leader to prove she went. She tells me she just keeps forgetting to have him sign. And then there are the urines. She's supposed to be getting regular tox screens on her urine to prove that she's clean. She did a few in the beginning but hasn't done any now in three months. First she said it was because she didn't have health insurance, but I called and they said that she didn't need to have insurance. When I told her that she said she hadn't known. Now, she mostly says that Timothy was too sick and she couldn't leave him to go give the urine samples."

"I don't know what to say. Like I said, I haven't seen her myself in a while. I did see Barbara and Jamal just now, outside the clinic."

"How did they seem? I haven't been able to see them in more than a month—sometimes they are in the apartment when I come over, but the grandmother never lets me stay if Joan's not around."

"They seemed okay, I guess. Barbara was a little strange . . ."

"What do you mean?"

"Oh, I don't know. Maybe it was nothing. Listen, Timothy has an appointment with me this afternoon. I'll talk to Joan then. I'll try to find out what's going on."

"Great. Thanks."

Timothy was my first patient of the afternoon.

"I been giving him the nebs, and they help for a while, but before long he's wheezing again."

Timothy was almost a year old; it startled me to see how different he was from the last time I'd seen him. He was big, and chubby, with a wild Afro. I ran my fingers through his hair and smiled.

"I know," said Joan. "I need to cut it or braid it. I keep meaning to do one or the other, but I guess I kind of like it this way."

I listened to his chest as he sat on Joan's lap. He was wheezing, although not very badly.

"When did you last give him a neb?" I asked.

"Oh, about two hours ago," said Joan. She looked thinner than I remembered her, but other than that she looked exactly the same.

"He doesn't sound terrible, but he doesn't sound good, either. We'll give him another neb here, and then I think it would help if he took some steroids for a few days."

I sat down on the chair at the desk, next to them.

"How have you been while I was gone?" I asked.

"Okay, I guess," she said with a shrug.

"What happened with the GED program?" Before I left, she had been excited about getting her high school diploma.

Joan sighed. "Didn't work out," she said. "I kept missing classes 'cause of Timothy's asthma. I dropped out."

"Couldn't your mother take care of him?"

"Sometimes she can. But she gets real tired real easily, and sometimes takin' care of Timothy is just too much for her. Besides, she smokes, and that makes him wheeze even worse."

She shifted Timothy from one knee to the other. "I want to get a job, you know, so that I can move out, get my own place, buy things for my kids. But I'd just be missin' it 'cause of Timothy. And even if he stopped wheezing for a while, I'd have to pay for child care 'cause I couldn't leave him with my mother all the time with her health problems and her smoking, and there's no way no job I could get is gonna pay enough for child care and insurance and still have enough for food and rent."

"What about day care vouchers? Can't you get those when you go off welfare?"

"For a while, I think. But then you're on your own and then I'd end up quitting. I think it's better if I go to school first, then I could get a better job. That's what I'm gonna do, as soon as I can. Soon as Timothy's a little bigger and his asthma's a little better, that's what I'm gonna do."

She said this with certainty. Timothy coughed.

"Oh, the neb," I said. "Sorry, Timothy." I got the oxygen tank and tubing, and reached for the medication and saline that were on the table.

"I can do it," said Joan. She took the medication, measured it out perfectly into the cup, added the saline, and attached the clear plastic mask. I turned the oxygen on as she carefully fastened the mask onto Timothy's face.

"You do a good job," I said, sitting down again.

She smiled. "I get lots of practice," she said. "I spend a lot of the day sittin' in our bedroom, doing this. I keep him in the bedroom whenever I'm in there, to keep him away from the cigarette smoke."

"It must be hard to keep him in there all the time, though—I mean, like when you're doing housework or stuff."

"I don't really do any of that stuff," she said, laughing. "Me and my kids, we're mostly in the bedroom. We even eat in there. I got an old TV there for me and the kids to watch. So I figure that I just gotta keep that clean. I do the bathroom sometimes, but nothin' else. My mother, she does the cleaning."

"What about shopping?"

Joan looked at me sideways, clearly wondering why I was asking. I kept my face blank.

"She does the shopping, too. I give her my food stamps and WIC stuff."

She seemed to have more energy than she did the last time I saw her, but it was a nervous energy. She talked faster, her voice was sharper, she sat more upright in the chair than she used to.

"How are the NA meetings going?"

"Oh, great," she said immediately.

"Any trouble getting to them, what with the kids and all?"

"No, no trouble."

"Must be hard sometimes, when Barbara and Jamal need help with their homework."

"Oh, they never need help. They do fine all by themselves."

I wanted to scream at her, I wanted to shake her. Yet I was afraid to betray Barbara—I didn't know what the consequences would be for her. And, more important, I really wanted Joan to tell me herself.

"Staying clean must be a real challenge sometimes with the stresses of raising three kids."

She looked at me sideways again. Her eyes were alert, but a little unfocused. "It's not so bad," she said.

There was no reason for her to tell me if she was using drugs again, I realized. There was no reason for her to tell me anything except what she thought I wanted to hear. I had nothing to offer her, at least nothing that she wanted. I couldn't take care of Timothy or pay for his child care. I couldn't get her an apartment or make it possible for her to get a well-paying job. I could offer her drug treatment options, but they had been offered to her already. Her decisions and her reasons were not things I could touch—she did not know me or trust me enough for that.

And if she told me that she was using drugs again, I might call DSS. I would have to, really, unless I felt that the children were in no danger; as a pediatrician, I was a "mandated reporter," obliged by law to report abuse or neglect. Joan had already shown that she didn't care for the children well when she was using; there was no reason to think it would be any different now. And if I called DSS, they might take the children away.

The only noise in the room was the soft hiss of the oxygen bubbling through the medication. Timothy sat calmly on Joan's lap, breathing in the mist in the mask, looking at me and the room and Joan, who was looking at her shoes.

It is strange how so often even though we are right next to someone, we might as well be on opposite sides of the earth.

"Yeah," Joan said, more softly and without looking up, "that's what I'm gonna do. Soon's I can, I'm gonna go to school and then I'll get a good job and me and the kids'll move to our own place. Everything will be fine then."

I didn't say anything; in that moment, I couldn't say anything. I turned to Timothy's chart and wrote down what his chest had sounded like and how much medication we had given him. I turned back and checked the chamber below the mask to see if the medication was finished. It was, so I turned off the oxygen and gently took the mask off Timothy's face. He was breathing more comfortably, and when I listened to his chest with my stethoscope I didn't hear any more wheezing.

I wrote out the prescription for the steroids and handed it to her. "Give him half a teaspoon, twice a day, in the morning and at bedtime, for five days. Do the nebs four times a day, at least for the next week or so. Call us if he gets any worse or if he doesn't start to get much better in a day or two." My tone was abrupt and businesslike. She nodded. I got up and walked to the door. I was just about out when I turned around.

"Call if you need anything, if there's anything at all we can do, okay?" I said, almost pleading.

"Okay," she said distractedly as she picked Timothy up with one arm and picked the diaper bag up with the other. Timothy grinned at me and waved bye-bye.

I watched her go out the swinging doors to the lobby. Sarah came up behind me, watching her too.

"I remember her so well as a little girl," she said. "She was so full of spunk. Everyone used to say that she was going to be something when she grew up—go to college, be something. She liked it when people said that. 'I'm gonna be something!' she'd say, and we all used to think it was cute."

"So why'd she quit school?" I asked, still staring at Joan, who was making her way somewhat clumsily to one of the chairs in the waiting room.

"I think because she had to, or at least because she thought she had to. And I'm sure she never thought it would be a problem to go back."

Joan picked up Timothy's coat from the floor where she had dropped it along with everything else when she sat down. She stood Timothy up on the floor, leaning him against her knees for support, and started putting the coat on him.

The doors to the outside opened with a rush of cold air, and in came Barbara and Jamal, laughing and covered with snow.

"Hey, Mama, look at us!" said Jamal brightly. "We're snowmen!"

"Yeah, whatever," said Joan, not looking up.

They both stopped laughing. Barbara bent down and started to help with Timothy's coat, putting in on and zipping it up under and around Joan's hands.

Jamal stood there for a moment, watching. Then he turned and he was gone, with the door closing softly behind him.

Sixteen

There are days at Martha Eliot when I speak almost no English at all. In a morning of seeing ten to twelve patients for well child care it's not uncommon that I'll have only one or two with English-speaking families, and sometimes none of the families speak English. And often the nursing assistant I'm working with is Marta, who tends to speak to me in Spanish too. I don't mind, actually; it is simpler to stay in one language.

By the end of some days I am thinking in Spanish. I'll turn on the radio in the car as I'm leaving, and it will take me a few minutes to understand what the people are saying. Or I'll stop by the drugstore on the way home and feel disoriented by the fact that the other customers aren't speaking Spanish. I feel like I'm in the wrong country.

But I'm not, of course. I'm in the United States, and in certain pockets and places in the United States one hears very little English.

I'm not sure of the immigration status of all the Latino children I see. The majority are citizens, having been born here. But many were not born here; they were born elsewhere and usually raised initially by their extended family, joining their parents in the United States after the parents can manage to care for them. Some of the children have all the appropriate papers to be here—or at least had the papers at some point—and some of them don't.

The immigration status of the parents can be much murkier. I know many families who have gone about everything to the letter of the law, and I know others who haven't. I've actually stopped asking specific questions about this unless I need to know, like when I'm trying to get specific services for a family, or when I'm making plans for a child that would have to be changed if they might imminently be leaving the country. Otherwise, I keep my questions limited. I am a pediatrician, not a representative of the INS.

Recently, though, I have been thinking about asking more questions about status—not to report people, but to warn them.

There is an anti-immigration and anti-immigrant swell in this country that is growing. There is much complaining about the money that immigrants, legal and illegal, cost taxpayers. There are accusations that immigrants steal jobs and therefore livelihood from those born here. There are all sorts of plans. Some are relatively mild, like increasing border controls, but others are more extreme, like denying benefits to legal immigrants until they have worked and contributed to the tax base for ten years, or denying citizenship to babies of noncitizens who are born in this country. The rhetoric seems to be growing stronger, and I am puzzled and troubled by the anger it expresses.

I can't argue with the fact that immigrants, especially illegal immigrants, cost taxpayers money. Health care is expensive. Schooling is expensive, too; I'm sure that it costs the taxpayers a reasonable amount of money every year to provide education and special services for noncitizen children.

Lots of immigrants I've seen have come to the United States for really good reasons, such as escaping persecution or deep, terrible poverty. But some clearly do come, often illegally, with plans to get a least some of their income from the government. They admit it openly.

This doesn't make me angry, because I don't blame them—why *not* move from a situation of poverty and poor resources where you have to work your fingers to the bone for very little money into a situation where you can get a check from the government twice a month and have access to good health care and services? It is, however, unfair to those who do things legally—and it does make me uncomfortable that it is apparently so easy for people to move in and out of this country illegally. So while I think we need to be careful to put in place exceptions for people who come here illegally to escape persecution or death, I think it would be a good idea to try to do a better job of controlling illegal immigration.

But the talk about cutting benefits to legal immigrants who are disabled or who haven't been working here very long is mean-spirited, I think, and hypocritical. Except for Native Americans, we are all immigrants. If we are not ourselves fresh from another country, we are the descendants of immigrants, who came in pursuit of opportunity and a better life, some of whom were in need of help. Maybe they didn't get a government subsidy, because they didn't have such things at the time, but somebody may have offered them a place to live, or food, or clothing, or found them a job. This is our history; we are the country of "the golden door" lit by the Statue of Liberty's lamp. Maybe the golden door is closing—but then we need to recognize that that is what we are doing as a country, and face what it means about us.

The talk about cutting or refusing benefits to the children of immigrants is much more disturbing. The children did not do anything wrong; the decisions were made by someone else, and they are simply living them out. They do not deserve to be hungry, or ill, or robbed of the future an education could give them.

If you cut benefits to the children of immigrants, I hear the politicians say, then you decrease the incentives for illegal immigration. I suppose that's true, but as someone who looks every day into the faces of those children, I know it's not right.

Rosa, who is twelve, was born with a rare disease that slowly and progressively causes damage to almost every part of her body. Already, her growth is poor—she is the size of a six-year-old—and her weak muscles make it hard for her to climb the stairs at school. Her eyes are affected; she can barely move them and her eyelids do not close well. She has hormonal problems, for which she must take medications, and there are signs that her heart is not functioning as well as it should.

Rosa is full of smiles and hugs for us whenever she comes to the clinic. She draws us beautiful pictures, and ignores with grace the comments her size and appearance bring from people in the waiting room; she has a strong, proud spirit. She is a bright child who does well in school, but we do not know how long this will last, for a recent CAT scan of her brain showed that it is beginning to be affected. We do not know how long she will live, either—but we do know that the resources and medicines necessary to care for her would be essentially impossible to find in the Dominican Republic, where her family emigrated from, legally. The only way the family can afford those resources and medicines here is with the help of Rosa's Social Security disability benefits, for the small grocery the family runs generates only a meager income. If Rosa could not get those benefits any longer, or if her family had to return to the Dominican Republic, the effect on Rosa would be devastating and probably fatal.

Javier is eight, with shaggy dark hair and shy eyes. He is healthy, but there is something wrong with him. He didn't say anything at all until he was three, and he still doesn't put sentences together well. He has trouble following instructions, cannot write letters or numbers, and has difficulty remembering even simple things.

His hearing and vision are normal. His intelligence is actually normal, too. What the teachers at his school think is that he has a severe learning disability. He is in a special, small class for children with this kind of problem, and he is making progress. It is slow progress, but the teachers are optimistic that with time and lots of specialized attention he will learn to read and write. He and his mother are illegal immigrants from a small village in the Dominican Republic. It's unlikely that he would get any specialized attention there, or any chance at a future beyond menial labor.

Certainly Rosa and Javier are extremes, and perhaps we could legislate exceptions for children such as them. Or, perhaps they are not our responsibility at all, and we do not have to be concerned about them.

Perhaps none of them are our responsibility, none of the dark-haired, dark-eyed children who fill the waiting room at Martha Eliot, whose voices with their mixture of Spanish and English fill the air. Then it would not be our obligation to teach them to read—or to teach them anything, for that matter. We would not have to worry if they will get antibiotics for their ear infections and their pneumonias, or medications to help them breathe when their asthma attacks. It would not be our concern if their stomachs rumble empty all day and they grow thin and weak. It would not be our duty to stop them from living in subway tunnels, with nothing to keep them warm in winter's bitter cold. It would not be our problem if they die.

But it *would* be our problem. It may be true that these children shouldn't be here but they *are* here, and no amount of rhetoric will erase their needs. If we choose to abdicate our responsibility for them, we are choosing to be a society that knowingly and actively harms children.

I think that this is what it all gets down to, really: choosing our values as a society. We must be very careful as we do so; we must remember that our decisions leave a legacy, that they are examples for the generations that will follow.

Seventeen

The eardrum was clear and grayish, like a tiny piece of waxed paper, and when I squeezed the rubber ball attached with tubing to the otoscope, it moved briskly back and forth in response to the puff of air.

The antibiotics had cured the ear infection. *"No hay más infección,"* I said to Señora Gonzalez, who nodded. She had told me that the infection was gone; she knew Eliana was better.

Eliana Molina smiled a toothy wet smile at me. She hadn't cried at all while I examined her, another sign that she was feeling better. She sat in Señora Gonzalez's lap, a chubby little Buddha-child dressed all in pink with a pink headband peeking out from her dark curls. She was a year old now; Señora Gonzalez had brought pictures of the birthday party to show me.

I sat down at the desk to look at them, picture after slightly out-of-focus picture of the children posing or in motion, of the birthday banner and the big birthday cake with FELIZ CUMPLEAÑOS ELIANA written on it in pink frosting.

"Fue de chocolate," said Carlos. His voice was still soft but stronger than before. His hair was neatly trimmed, and his eyes were bright. Sharina sat next to him in the chair, holding the same doll that Marta had given her on her first visit to the clinic. She had grown quite a bit since I last saw her, and looked very healthy. Her eyes were still as big as saucers, but they had lost the shell-shocked sheen they used to have.

"Yeah, and it was the worst chocolate cake I ever had," said Daisy. She sat in the other chair I'd brought in, next to Carlos and Sharina.

Señora Gonzalez shot her a frowning glance.

"That's not very nice, Daisy," I said. "I'm sure that Señora Gonzalez worked hard on that cake."

Daisy put her chin in the air and looked at me sideways, blankly. "Well, it was bad," she said.

"It was good," said Carlos quietly, staring angrily at Daisy. He was clearly more comfortable with English now, and I wondered how much it was from speaking English in arguments with Daisy.

Señora Gonzalez's deep, firm voice intervened, speaking to me. *"¿Y Carlos, puede Ud. chequiarlo?"* She had asked me if I would check Carlos too, as he had been complaining of a stomachache.

I motioned Carlos up onto the table. He smiled, jumped up, and let me help him off with his shirt without hesitation. He was still very thin, but he looked stronger. He answered my questions in Spanish, quickly and seriously. It hurt him in the middle of his stomach, he said, but not really anymore. No, he didn't feel like throwing up. No, he hadn't had any diarrhea, and he wasn't having trouble going to the bathroom, either.

I asked him to lie down on the table and he did, still smiling at me. I felt his stomach with my right hand, pushing in to check for any tenderness, or a big liver or spleen, or anything else. He squirmed a little, smiling.

"¿Te da cosquillas?" I asked—does it tickle? He nodded, and giggled.

I told Señora Gonzalez that he seemed fine, that whatever had been giving him the stomachache probably wasn't serious, but that she should call if the pain came back.

"Maybe he was just pretending to be sick," said Daisy.

"Was not," said Carlos.

"I'm sure he was sick," I said. "He's just better today."

"He's a little liar," said Daisy.

"¡Daisy!" said Señora Gonzalez sharply. Daisy folded her arms in front of her and moved to a corner of the room, where she stood sullenly, leaning against the wall.

* * *

"I can't get to Daisy at all," Sara Daviles, the psychologist, had told me. "She just sits there and won't say anything except insulting remarks about me or the Gonzalez family or her siblings—about everything, really. She's been coming just about every week for months now, and she won't even begin to open up, no matter how hard I try with her."

She sat back in her chair, pensive, her right index finger playing with the corner of her glasses. Then she leaned forward again. "It's a problem, too, because she's doing stuff that is worrisome. First there was the fire—"

"The fire?" I interrupted. "She set a fire?"

"Well, said Sara, "we don't know for sure. She said it was an accident, that she was just looking at the cigarette lighter and didn't expect it to light, and that when it did she was startled and she dropped it on the pile of newspaper in the kitchen by accident. Carlos said she was lying, that she had talked about setting a fire, but nobody was in the room with her when it happened so there's no way to really know."

"Was anybody hurt?"

"No, no. Luckily, Señor Gonzalez came in right as the newspapers started to burn, and he put the fire out before there was much to it. He said that Daisy was just standing there looking at it."

"She didn't call for help?"

"No, she didn't. When I asked her why she said it was because she was scared, which is a reasonably good excuse, so I didn't push it. But then a week or so later she pulled a knife on one of the Gonzalez's teenage sons."

"She didn't really," I gasped.

Sara smiled at the expression on my face. "She absolutely did," she said.

"But why? What was he doing to her?"

"Nothing, apparently. They don't like each other, that's clear—

but he says that he just avoids her, and Señora Gonzalez confirms this. He seems like an honest, reliable kid, too, so I believe what he says. He said that he was in the kitchen eating breakfast and Daisy came up behind him with a carving knife and held it next to his neck. She says that she was just playing, but he said that it didn't seem like she was playing. He said that the way she looked at him was terrifying."

"What did he do?"

"Nothing. He was too scared. He just sat there, and after a few seconds she laughed and put the knife away and said that he better watch out for her."

"I'd be really nervous having Daisy in my home," I said. "I admire Señora Gonzalez."

"She *is* nervous. Very nervous, actually. I talked with her about having Daisy moved to a specialized foster home, one for kids with behavioral problems. But she wants to keep the kids together. She says that after everything they've been through it would be too hard on them to separate them. She really wants to help them; I think she has grown really fond of them. She has even talked about adopting all four, but Daisy may just sabotage that if she doesn't stop."

"They're free for adoption?"

"No, not yet. The mother is in jail. The DA came down hard on her, got her for aggravated assault or something like that. DSS is working to get her to terminate her parental rights, and it's looking like that will happen. The father of Sharina and Eliana was picked up on various drug charges and has agreed to terminate his parental rights as part of a plea bargain. The father of Daisy and Carlos is in Puerto Rico and has made some noises about trying to get custody, but nobody thinks he will follow through on it. He hasn't seen the kids or been involved at all since shortly after Carlos was born."

"Has Daisy been this way all along?"

"Yeah, more or less. Señora Gonzalez says that she was hard to manage from the start. But things have gotten worse since their mother was sent to jail. Daisy and Carlos saw it in the newspaper. Señora Gonzalez didn't realize the story was going to be there, and they got to the paper before she did. The next day was the incident with Daisy and the fire."

Sara sighed, a long, sad sigh. "Daisy makes me feel so frustrated, so helpless. She is always just out of my reach. I've never met a kid who made me feel so helpless."

Daisy stood out of reach, in the corner, watching me distrustfully as I helped Carlos put his shirt back on.

"How's school?" I asked him.

"I like it," he said. "My teacher is nice."

"Are you learning a lot?"

"I'm trying," he said seriously. "But I'm not very smart."

"El es uno de los mejores estudiantes en su clase," said Señora Gonzalez—Carlos was one of the best students in his class. Carlos blushed, and climbed down from the table. Señora Gonzalez motioned to him; he went over to her. She moved Eliana to one knee and wrapped her free arm around Carlos. He laughed and wriggled out from under her arm, going back to sit on his chair.

Daisy was having a lot of problems in school, Señora Gonzalez told me. The teachers said that she was very smart, but she was lazy. As Señora Gonzalez said this, Daisy looked at her angrily. Señora Gonzalez looked back at Daisy sadly, then turned to me.

"Pero ella baila muy bien," she said—but she dances very well. Looking back at Daisy every few seconds, she told me how the school had put on a holiday pageant and Daisy had danced a solo piece. Everyone thought it was beautiful. She was hoping that they could find a way to afford to send Daisy to dance class, because she was very talented.

Slowly, a smile spread over Daisy's face, and her arms unfolded, moving down to her sides.

"Would you show me, Daisy?" I asked. "Could I see some of your dance?"

Daisy hesitated, and then said, "Well, okay, just a little." She came out of the corner into the center of the room. She held her arms up above her, elegantly, and did a pirouette. Then she took took two delicate tiptoe steps and dipped down with one leg out straight behind her, toes pointed, holding it for a few seconds and then bringing herself upright again into another pirouette. She moved as if weightless, in perfect form.

"Daisy, that was beautiful," I said. "How did you learn to do that?"

"From TV," she said. "I watched people dance on TV."

"I was in the show too," said Carlos eagerly.

Daisy whirled around to face him. "Yeah, you were just a candy cane. Anybody could be a candy cane."

Carlos's face fell.

"Daisy, be nice!" said Sharina, stamping her foot.

I was stunned. "She talked!" I said.

Daisy shrugged. "She's been doing that for a while," she said.

"Nobody told me. When did she start? *¿Cuando empezó a hablar?*"

Sharina had started about two months before, Señora Gonzalez told me. One day, completely unexpectedly, she started talking— in full sentences. She mostly spoke English; Señora Gonzalez wasn't sure why. She still didn't talk very often.

"She only talks when she feels like it," said Carlos proudly.

I knelt down next to Sharina. Her hair had grown longer and Señora Gonzalez had it braided in two short braids tied with blue ribbon. She wore a red-and-blue-checked dress, blue tights, and shiny black shoes. She stood straight and defiant, smiling at me.

"You have a lovely voice," I said to her. "Do you like talking?"

She shrugged.

"What do you like?" I asked.

"I like cookies."

I laughed. "Me too. What else?"

"I like my bed. It is big and warm."

This time Señora Gonzalez laughed. *"¿Si te gusta tanto tu cama, porqué te encuentro todas las noches en la cama de Carlos?"*—if you like your bed so much, why do I find you every night in Carlos's bed?

Every night it was the same, Señora Gonzalez told me. She'd put Sharina to sleep in her own bed, but in the middle of the night Sharina would get up and go into Carlos's room and climb in bed with him. She didn't wake him; she would just curl up by his feet.

"Why, Sharina?" I asked. "Why do you go to Carlos's bed?"

Sharina shrugged. "Because I miss him," she said matter-of-factly. Then she turned, with an air of regal dismissiveness, and went back to the chair. She slid up again next to Carlos and hugged her doll.

Eliana had been trying to get down off Señora Gonzalez's lap. Señora Gonzalez let her, and she worked her way down toward Carlos and Sharina unsteadily, holding on carefully to Señora Gonzalez's coat and then Carlos's knee. When she got to Sharina she reached for Sharina's doll, grabbing a fist full of the doll's bright yellow hair.

"No!" yelled Sharina. "Mine!"

This startled Eliana, who let go of Carlos's knee and began to fall backward. She held on even more tightly to the doll's hair, pulling on it to regain her balance, and suddenly the doll's head popped off and Eliana fell down onto her bottom with the doll's head in her hand.

There was a brief silence, and then Daisy and Carlos started to laugh. They began at precisely the same moment, and this seemed to make them laugh even more. They looked at each other and their whole faces lit up with their laughter. Daisy sat back down on the chair and she and Carlos leaned together over Sharina, until their heads were touching.

Sharina's face was very red, and tears started to stream down her cheeks.

"Oh, honey," I said, "don't cry—*no llores*. We can fix it. It's an easy thing to fix, don't worry."

Señora Gonzalez scooped the startled Eliana up off the floor, dusting off her bottom, and putting her back on her lap. Gently, she took the doll's head out of Eliana's still clenched fist. She held her hand out to Sharina for the doll's body. Tentatively, Sharina lay the doll in Señora Gonzalez's hand. She climbed down off the chair and went to Señora Gonzalez. Sharina leaned against her and looked up at her with wide and tearful eyes.

Carefully and firmly, Señora Gonzalez pushed the doll's head back onto its body. "*Sí,*" she said. "*Esto puedo hacer*"—this I can do.

Eighteen

Kevin was admitted to the hospital almost monthly for a while after that first hospitalization. It was always the same thing: he would have a fever, for no apparent reason, and we would have to admit him to give him antibiotics intravenously for a couple of days while we waited for the results of the blood culture, which were always negative.

It got to be that I could tell the moment I walked into the room that he had a fever and was going to be admitted from the way Luz would look up at me. I couldn't necessarily tell immediately from Kevin, for often he would be smiling and playing despite his fever. But Luz would look at me with heavy, sad eyes, and I would know.

She began to get used to the hospital and its routines; with each admission she seemed a little less scared and overwhelmed. She never knew entirely what was going on because her English was so poor. She never asked for an interpreter, despite my repeated explanations of how available they were. She learned enough English to answer the doctors' and nurses' questions, which was easy, because they were always the same: questions about Kevin's symptoms, his previous hospitalizations, and his medications. Because she could answer these, albeit in broken, incorrect English, often people at the hospital would assume she spoke it well and rattle off explanations and instructions in English, leaving her in the dust after the first sentence.

She stayed with Kevin every moment, and mostly kept him in her arms. She'd sit with him in the chair during the day, and then at night she would unfold the chair into a cot and lay Kevin next to her there. She waited until he was in a deep sleep to use the bath-room or shower or run down to the cafeteria for food.

She told me one time when I came to visit that Kevin was mostly in her arms at home, too. She had a crib for him, a second-hand one she had bought from a friend. There was just enough room in her bedroom, she said, to wedge it between the bed and the wall. But she didn't like to leave him in it for long; he looks so small and alone there, she said.

Luz had a one-bedroom apartment in Roxbury, at the back of the second floor of a two-family house. The owner had made an extra apartment to increase his income. He divided two rooms off the rest of the second floor, put a small electric stove and a refrigerator in one of the rooms, and put a shower stall into what had been a half-bath. The only sink was in the bathroom, so that's where she washed her dishes. The entrance was off a rickety porch that she reached by squeezing past the garbage cans and climbing up even more rickety stairs.

Ricardo paid half of the rent; otherwise, Luz said, the rent would have taken up most of her welfare check. As it was, after utilities, there wasn't much left each month. Ricardo gave her money for clothes for the baby and sometimes bought diapers for him, too, which helped.

Her voice rose and fell musically as she spoke, although she always spoke softly, obviously made self-conscious by the family on the other side of the curtain in the semiprivate room and the nurses and other hospital staff who frequently walked through. She seemed like a shy person, yet she was eager to talk to me, maybe because nobody else spoke Spanish, maybe because of loneliness.

In the Dominican Republic she had been a hairdresser, and her dream had been to come to the United States and open up her own shop. She'd heard all the stories about everybody being able to make money here—even without working. If you can't find a job, her friends told her, the government will still pay you.

She was sad about being on welfare. It wasn't what she had wanted, she told me. She hadn't meant to get pregnant. She was going to make it on her own, and then maybe get married and have children. But Ricardo, he really wanted her to have a baby. She tried to be careful and not get pregnant, but it happened anyway.

I asked why Ricardo couldn't support her more, help pay for day care and other expenses so that she could get a job and get off welfare. It seemed only fair, since it was his idea to have Kevin.

Her face took on a dark blankness and she shook her head. He gave her things, she said; he helped. She didn't want to ask him for more. And as she always did when I brought up Ricardo, she changed the subject.

I liked being with Luz. I was always late for work when I went to see Kevin in the hospital, because I would end up staying to talk and the time would go by before I realized it. There was something about her that intrigued me and put me at ease. Her stories drew me in, and she didn't seem intimidated by me the way so many other mothers were. She would laugh with me, tell jokes, roll her eyes about something someone said or did. She listened to what I said about Kevin's condition, but unlike other mothers who just sat there nodding while I spoke, Luz always had questions and suggestions.

She asked about my children all the time. Early on she had looked at the rings on my finger and asked if I had children. Yes, I'd told her, and one of them is a little boy who is just a month older than Kevin. So we began to share stories about our sons, stories of their births and first smiles, stories of watching them while they slept and of imagining the men they would become.

Luz's hair and makeup were always neatly done. Usually her hair was pulled back in a simple knot, although sometimes she did it in many braids and then wound the braids together at the nape of her neck. Her clothes were not expensive, but they were always clean and pressed. She was small, a little more than five feet tall, and lithe; she reminded me of a cat in the way she held herself and moved.

I never saw Ricardo in the hospital. He did come visit, Luz assured me. He was very concerned about Kevin. He came in the evenings, sometimes with his mother, who would hold Kevin and cry, which made Luz angry. She never offers to help, never even comes to visit when he's not in the hospital, she said—what right does she have to come now and cry?

I did see Ricardo at the clinic; he would drive Luz and Kevin over for visits. He never said much. If I addressed him directly, he would respond, and pleasantly, although his responses were very brief, as close to "yes" or "no" as possible. He generally spoke English with me, even when I spoke to him in Spanish. He was from the Dominican Republic as well, but he had grown up in the United States and so spoke English fluently. He worked as a deliveryman for a furniture store, and picked up extra hours some nights as a security guard through an agency, covering people's vacations and sick days. He told me all this reluctantly, as if he didn't like to give out any details about himself.

Luz was quieter when Ricardo was there. She still asked questions and made suggestions, but she was briefer and more muted. She turned to look at him frequently, as if looking for his reaction; usually I didn't see any, but I could tell that Luz did sometimes by the way she'd pause and change the direction of what she was saying.

Sometimes when Ricardo touched her Luz seemed uncomfortable, although it was subtle and I wasn't sure. Other times when he touched her she would smile at him, a sweet, tender, slightly flirtatious smile. Always, she seemed in awe of him.

Ricardo obviously doted on Kevin. Once he got to know me a little I could always get a smile from him for saying something, anything, positive about Kevin, which was easy to do. As he grew, he became more and more beautiful: his hair grew in thick and curly, his eyes sparkled, and he had a smile that was heartwarming and heartbreaking at the same time. He stayed small for his age but he gained weight, filling out his cheeks and adding some fat under the smooth chocolate-colored skin of his legs. He was precocious; at nine months he was on the verge of walking, and although he couldn't talk he clearly understood a great deal. He watched his mother carefully, smiled when she smiled, and stopped smiling the moment she stopped. He watched me with wariness and curiosity, willing to play with me but only if he was in Luz's arms. He smiled at Ricardo and would go to him if Ricardo held out his arms, but Kevin didn't seem to like to be in Ricardo's arms for long. Soon he would be wriggling and reaching for Luz.

It was heartbreaking to see Kevin's confusion in the hospital, the way he stared at his IV, cowered from the doctors and nurses, and cried bitterly when he had blood drawn. He was too young to explain anything to, of course. But even if he had been old enough, there was no good explanation, not really.

One day Luz and Kevin came alone. It was a routine visit, for an immunization. Luz seemed distracted. And for the first time since I'd met her, she looked disheveled: her hair was loose, she wore no makeup, her clothes were wrinkled.

I asked if something was wrong, but she shook her head and said that everything was fine.

Kevin was well and growing. I showed Luz his growth chart but instead of grinning as she usually would, she just nodded. She had no questions or suggestions this time.

I gave him his shot, in his leg even though he was starting to walk, because his arm still seemed too small to stick a needle into. He screamed and screamed, clinging to Luz.

Luz began to cry. A single tear glided down her dark cheek, and then suddenly there were many tears and she was sobbing. It startled Kevin, who stopped crying and stared at her.

I got the other chair and sat down close to her, putting my hand on her shoulder. I said that I wished she would tell me what was wrong, that it had to be more than just the shot. There may be something I can do, I said to her. Please trust me.

She took some deep breaths, slowly pushing back the sobs, and wiped her cheeks with the back of her hand.

"*Es Ricardo,*" she said.

"*¿Ricardo?*" I said. "*¿Le pasó algo?*"—did something happen to him?

She shook her head, fighting back more sobs. New tears started to fall. Kevin's hands went to her face, as if to catch them. Luz leaned over and kissed his head, then looked up and straight at me.

Ricardo pulled a knife on her, she said. They'd been having an argument; Luz had seen him with another woman, and she'd confronted him. He took a knife out of his pocket, opened it, and held the point at her cheek. He told her that the other woman was none of her business and that if she tried to tell him what to do he would cut her face, or worse. He held the knife there for a long time, and then he left.

Shivers ran up my spine.

I asked if he had ever done anything like that before. She hesitated. He hadn't pulled a knife on her before, she said. But he had hit her. Most of the time, he was nice to her. But sometimes he would get mad at her for something she said or something she did or something she wore and he would hit her.

I apologized for not seeing the bruises, for not knowing sooner. He was careful, she told me. He hit her in places where he knew her clothes would hide the bruises.

Anger and fear welled up inside me. I said that she needed to get a restraining order. "*Estás en peligro*"—you're in danger.

She sighed, and looked away. She said softly that she didn't think he would do anything really bad to her. He was not a bad man. He loved her. And she loved him.

"*¿Si te quiere, porqué te hace todo esto?*"—if he loves you, why does he do all this to you?

She shrugged. Because I make him angry, she said.

"*No, no, no,*" I said, touching her shoulder again. "*El amor no es así*"—that's not the way love is.

"*A veces es así,*" she said—sometimes it is.

"*Mereces mejor,*" I said—you deserve better.

She shrugged again. Besides, she said, sitting up straighter, she needed him. Without the money he gave her each month, she couldn't afford the apartment. She needed a home for her son.

I asked if there was anyone, anyone at all, she could live with. She said that she had a sister in Boston, but her apartment was just as small as Luz's. She could stay there in an emergency for a few days, but she couldn't live there. She'd applied for public housing, but she was way at the bottom of a long waiting list.

I said that there were shelters for battered women and their children. From her reaction, I could tell that she had never thought of herself as a "battered woman." She looked down at the floor for a while and then said that she didn't want to be in a shelter with Kevin. They were too crowded. He would get sick.

I said that there were advocates for battered women at Children's Hospital, that there was someone we could call right then, together, who might be able to help.

She shook her head immediately and firmly. My response to the situation was clearly making her uncomfortable. It wasn't such a bad problem, she said. She would be okay. She could take care of herself and her son.

She started putting Kevin's clothes back on him.

I said that she would be safer with a restraining order.

"*Quizás,*" she said. "*Quizás no*"—maybe, maybe not.

She finished with the clothes. "*¿Eso es todo?*"

I sat in the chair, feeling helpless and stupid, and said that yes, that was all. I asked her to please think about the restraining order, and to please call, any time of night or day, if she needed help. I wrote my home phone number down on a piece of paper and handed it to her; she folded it carefully and put it in her purse.

She stood up with Kevin, putting her purse on her shoulder. She looked down at me, smiled briefly but genuinely, and walked out of the room to the lobby.

I sat there in a fog of emotion watching her go, full of swirling words that would not come together. I found myself wishing she would walk more carefully—pull Kevin in tighter, keep her steps long but narrow. The edge was terribly close.

Nineteen

I was becoming more and more distracted.

I would find myself standing in the middle of the kitchen, having forgotten what it was I went there to do. Or I'd be kneeling by the bathtub, filling it to bathe the children, and suddenly I'd realize it was about to overflow. Or I'd trail off at the end of a sentence while reading the children a story, realizing it only when Michaela tugged at my shirt.

There was no one particular thing on my mind. Some of it was to-do lists of household chores, bills to pay, things to buy—details that whirled and scattered in my head. Some of it was the clinic: images of patients, remembering things they'd said or I'd said, wondering if I'd forgotten to do something, hoping they were feeling better, thinking about other things I might do to help them.

But it was more, and different, than having my mind filled with images and to-do lists. I felt off-balance, uneasy. Something didn't feel right.

I tried not thinking. I tried getting lost in the work of being home. The tasks were relentless, beginning early and ending late. There were diapers to be changed, arms to be put through armholes in shirts that got too small quickly; there were bottles to be mixed, given, and washed, and Cheerios to be poured out into little bowls with Winnie the Pooh on them. There were counters and a high chair to be wiped clean, and clumps of cold, wet clothing to move from the washer to the dryer. There were rugs to be vacuumed, and vacuumed again, and toys to be retrieved from under the couch. It was easy to move from one task to another literally all day long—but although the tasks filled my hands they rarely filled my mind. I couldn't really get lost in them.

Getting lost in the children was easier. Zachary was almost a year old, blossoming from a colicky baby into a sweetly obstinate boy. He refused to crawl; instead, he would pull himself to standing and then scream until someone held his hands and helped him walk wherever he wanted to go. After months of baldness, he had finally grown soft, golden hair, and his chestnut eyes broke and won my heart time and time again. Michaela was two, full of new words and tantrums, with wispy light brown hair and my mother's green-gray eyes. She was a complex child, whose responses were surprising and yet deeply familiar, like looking in a mirror back in time.

They pulled every emotion out of me, every feeling possible. Not all of the feelings were positive; there were moments with the children that were filled with frustration, like when Michaela threw full-blown tantrums in the grocery store or Zachary refused to go back to sleep in the middle of the night when I was so tired I could barely sit up. Sometimes the frustration edged into anger as one of them did exactly what I'd just told him or her not to, and I'd yell and feel sorry and stupid afterward.

But mostly what I felt when I was with them was joy. I loved the silly games of patty-cake and hide-and-seek, and the tickling and playing with dolls under the kitchen table. I loved the hugs, and the kissing away of tears; I loved how their bodies were so often against mine, how they belonged there just as much as they had belonged inside me before they were born. The fact of their existence filled me with wonder, and their beauty left me speechless.

Their beauty terrified me sometimes. I felt utterly and irretrievably vulnerable to badness and to circumstances, the accidents of life. As a pediatrician who had trained in a tertiary-care hospital, I had seen what those circumstances could do . . . the little girl with the headache who was diagnosed with a brain tumor, the boy with the bruise who was found to have leukemia, all those children who fell into pools and drowned when their parents ran to answer the phone or didn't realize they'd slipped out the door . . . I would put myself in the place of those parents, and the pain and panic were more than I could bear.

This terror was part of my distractedness and unease. It had begun and grown since becoming a parent, but working at Martha Eliot had made it worse. The life of the inner city seemed so full of random badness that it undermined my ability to trust the world. A little boy in his Halloween costume was shot dead because he was standing on that particular piece of ground at that particular moment in time. Almost any piece of ground could be deadly, if you were there at that unpredictably wrong moment. Lives could be lost over a bracelet or a jacket. Children were born into hunger, or lived in homes filled with rats or cockroaches or drugs, innocent souls stumbling into places where nobody should ever be.

I'd known it was out there, this badness; anybody who ever picks up a paper or watches the news knows it's there. But since I'd started working at Martha Eliot more of the places where the bad things happened were places I knew, places I'd been, and sometimes the people they happened to were people I knew. Since I'd started working at the clinic it had all become terribly real, and terribly close.

Anything could happen. I felt this acutely, and it held me like a cold, tight hand. Cancer, accidents, violence—there was so much out there that could harm those I loved most or take them from me. Badness could be very random. The world was not safe and I could not make it safe, no matter how hard I tried.

I would wake up at night in a cold sweat, still in the hold of a blur of a nightmare about something horrible happening to my family. I would lie in bed until my heart stopped racing, curling up into the small of Mark's back, drawing comfort from his warmth.

Then I would steal out of bed to the children's room and lay my hand on their chests, to be sure that they were still breathing.

Which, of course, they were. The odds that they would just suddenly stop breathing and die were exceedingly small, as were the odds that they would get cancer or be gunned down. In general, the odds are with us as we raise our children. Usually they survive. We know this, and to make life bearable we commute it into a belief that we and those we love are somehow protected, that bad things happen to other people, not us. We begin to believe that we will get what we deserve.

But spending my days as a physician, and working at Martha Eliot, I could not escape the fact that what we deserve often has nothing to do with what happens to us. Life is not bound by rules of fairness.

On the way to the park with Michaela and Zachary I'd stare at the crisp white houses with their lush lawns and carefully weeded flower beds and I'd think of Bromley-Heath. I'd think of how bits of broken glass, clear and green and brown, shiny and dull, litter some of the walkways and places where children play. I'd think of all the old, dark brick and the cement and chain-link fences and the heavy metal doors leading into graffiti-covered hallways that echo and sometimes smell of urine.

Why was I raising my children in Melrose instead of Bromley-Heath? The easy answer was that it was because I had earned it, through years of study and hard work. But I found that this answer didn't hold up well to close scrutiny. Yes, I had studied and worked hard. But so had my grandparents and then my parents, who had earned enough money to buy a house in a suburb with excellent public schools and pay for my accomplished and expensive education. That I be highly educated was their central dream for me, the dream they demandingly and persistently pursued until I pursued it too. My study and hard work began at a particular place, and that place where I began had everything to do with where I finished.

I know a young girl growing up in Bromley-Heath who wants to be a lawyer. She is certainly smart enough; she is bright and quick-witted, and so wise that it is startling that she is only fourteen. Her mother grew up on welfare and is on welfare herself but is determined to get off, determined that her four children will support themselves and make their way well in the world. She keeps them off the street, makes sure the children do their homework, keeps in close touch with the school. She studies with her children, taking courses at the community college, setting an example and gaining skills to get a job when the baby goes to school. The father doesn't help. He never has.

Their apartment is bright and cheery and clean, a fortress against the loud hallways and the gunshots and the groups of young men who move confidently in the night or the wild-eyed men and women moving in and out of doorways.

The mother's work shows in her daughter, who stands straight with shining brown eyes, who gets all A's, who is soft-spoken, polite, and optimistic. But if the girl is to be a lawyer, it will take more than that. She will have to fight for a good education in the stressed Boston public schools with their limited resources and teachers who have to do so much more than just teach. She will have to be strong against the pressures of her peers, many of whom will drift into gangs and drugs and pregnancy; they will play proud and pull at her, taunt her for being different. And if she can indeed fight and stay strong and keep getting A's and get accepted into college, she will have to find the crazy money it costs, competing for vanishing scholarships and signing her life away for the loan after loan it will take to cover expenses. Maybe she will be lucky and get a scholarship that lets her go away to college, but maybe she will only be able to afford to take courses at the community college and live at home, studying in her tiny shared bedroom in the housing development, making her way home at night past the young men and women on the corner who will say she thinks she's better than they, who will tease her and pull at her still. And if she can keep fighting, keep being strong and keep getting A's—then she will have to find a way to pay for law school.

Maybe she will pull it off. It's certainly possible; almost anything is possible. But it will take truly hard work, harder work than I ever faced, than my parents ever faced, than my children will probably ever face.

Most of the people in Bromley-Heath work hard. But place has power over lives. Much of the work of life in Bromley-Heath and the community around it goes into simply keeping one's head above water, into finding food and shelter and making some semblance of order within the chaos, into staying alive. Anything achieved beyond that, even if it's just avoiding bitterness, is impressive.

I had so very much, I would think sometimes as the bathtub threatened to overflow or Michaela tugged at my sleeve to finish the story. I had a place to live that was warm, dry, and secure. I had all sorts of possessions, like a car, a television, a VCR, a computer, a microwave. And I had two healthy children and a devoted, gentle, present husband. As I looked at it all I felt awkward, and guilty.

It was like a survivor's guilt. I was acutely aware that it was accident of birth, luck of the draw, as much as anything else that had brought me what I had. So I felt guilty—and terrified, because I knew that I had no real claim to what I had, and no real guarantee that I would keep any of it.

To fight the awful combination of guilt and terror, I found myself looking for things equally real that were comforting and good. I needed to find things that endured and that I could trust.

I began to see that the simplest things I did were perhaps the most real: baking bread, giving medications, mending clothes, feeding a baby, bandaging a wound, giving a hug. These things had intrinsic value, no matter what, and when the terror or the guilt began to creep in, I could draw the world down into simple things and take comfort in them.

If I concentrated on each child hot with fever under my stethoscope, each mother looking into my eyes, if I did my best to meet each need presented to me, I felt less guilty. If I concentrated on each meal to be prepared or shirt to be folded, each bath to be given, each lullaby to be sung— if I did my best to do them well and enjoy them, tomorrow's possibilities were less frightening.

I saw that relationships can be real, too. They may change, affected by circumstance and by mood, but the fact of them can endure—the fact of lives touching and mattering to each other. I felt strengthened by the number of lives that touched mine and comforted by knowing that there could always be more. I would always have my friendship and my commitment to offer. And while this couldn't wipe away differences and inequalities, it would always be worth something.

I still have the nightmares, and I still creep in to feel the rise and fall of my sleeping children's chests. But I am learning to take life one day, one task, one face at a time, and this helps. I'm learning, also, to appreciate deeply.

Twenty

S he's beautiful," I said.

Teresa grinned, and her eyes shone. "She is, ain't she," she said softly.

The baby on the exam table in front of me was two weeks old, and her name was Andrea. She was tiny and delicate, with a mop of wavy black hair, and round brown eyes. Her legs were very long for her little body; they reminded me of Lila's.

"She has long legs like you," I said to Lila, who was on her tip-toes standing close to me with her chin on the exam table, looking at the baby.

Lila looked up at me and smiled. "I'm her big sister," she said proudly. She was four years old now, taller and less skinny. She was dressed in jeans and a bright red shirt with flowers on it; the beads in her braids were yellow this time.

"You sure are," I said. "And I bet you're a really good one." Lila beamed.

I listened to Andrea's heart and lungs, felt her belly, checked her skin for rashes and birthmarks, looked in her eyes and ears and mouth, checked her reflexes.

I turned to Teresa. "She's absolutely perfect," I said as I swaddled the baby in a blanket and picked her up. "Can I hold her for a little while?"

"Sure," laughed Teresa. "I don't mind the break."

I sat down in the chair at the desk and cradled Andrea in my arms; she promptly fell asleep. Lila came over and leaned against my shoulder to see the baby's face.

"Lila, leave the doctor be," said Teresa. Her voice was less sharp than the one she used to use with Lila.

"I don't mind," I said. "Let her be a doting sister. Better that than jealous."

"True," said Teresa, readjusting herself in the chair.

"Are you okay?" I asked. "How are you feeling?"

"Not so bad," said Teresa. "I got a few stitches, still hurts a bit sometimes to sit on 'em. Labor was pretty quick, though, just about four hours. Easier than it was with Lila, that's for sure. She had me in labor for like twelve hours."

"You look good," I said. She did. She looked tired, which was to be expected, but her cheeks were full and rosy, her hair was neatly tucked under a bright blue scarf, and the blue sweatshirt and sweatpants she wore were clean. Her eyes were brighter than I'd seen them for a long time.

"Andrea has gained weight nicely," I said. "Are you breast-feeding?"

"I'm trying to do that some," she said, "but it's kind of hard. Sometimes it seems like she just don't want my breast—I think she likes the bottle better."

"Maybe because it's easier for her to get the milk out of the bottle than from your breast. But breast milk is better for her, if you can manage. Did you breast-feed the others at all?"

She shook her head. "I didn't want to—seemed like too much trouble. 'Sides, I was using, and I'd heard that the drugs could get into my milk, and I didn't want my babies to get no more drugs in 'em."

"I can't tell you how proud I am of you for not using," I said. "You must be proud, aren't you?"

She shrugged. "Not really," she said.

"Breast-feeding can be hard at the beginning," I said. "Do you have any friends who breast-feed, to help you out?"

She frowned at me. "No," she said, as if I'd just asked an absurd question.

"Well, do you at least have some family or friends around to take care of Lila and do housework for you so that you can really spend some time getting the breast-feeding right?"

She looked at me like I was from Mars. "No," she said. "There's people around, but they ain't helpful. But it's not so hard with Lila. She's in Head Start now every morning, and that gives me some time. She really likes it, too."

I turned to Lila. "So you like school?"

"I *love* school," said Lila. "I get to play and we make pictures. I eat breakfast there, too."

Her speech had improved dramatically, most probably because of school. She seemed more confident, too, and less desperate for attention.

I turned back to Teresa. "She looks great," I said, motioning toward Lila.

Teresa smiled proudly. "She's eatin' much better," she said. "She likes peanut butter so I make her lots of peanut butter sandwiches—you said they got lots of calories. She likes that milk shake stuff, too—that Carnation stuff that you said was good to give her. She been eatin' real good."

"Is she living with you more now?" I asked.

"I got custody of her now. Got all that stuff final a couple of months ago. My DSS worker, she thought I was ready, and Lila's daddy, well, he was gettin' tired of havin' to deal with her, so he didn't put up no fight."

I looked at Lila to see if she had any reaction to hearing this. She was busy kissing the baby's head; if she had a reaction, she didn't show it.

"He's Andrea's father, right?" She nodded. "Is he helping out? Is he visiting?"

Teresa sighed and leaned back in the chair. "Yeah, he visits, sometimes. He brings some money sometimes, too. I don't mind him visitin' sometimes—my girls should know their daddy. But I don't like him around too much."

Andrea stirred in my arms. I stroked her cheek and she went back to sleep.

"Why not?" I asked.

Teresa glanced over at Lila, who had wandered over to the window and was watching some men repair a fence.

"He's . . . well, he uses some, and here and there, well, I think he does some dealin'. He offers me stuff—I don't want that stuff 'round me, or's I might start wantin' it, y'know? 'Sides, he got bad friends, people I don't want in my place." She looked right at me as she spoke, her voice low but firm.

Andrea stirred again, opened her mouth wide and began to turn her head from side to side, whimpering a little.

"I think she's hungry," I said.

Teresa looked at the clock in the room. "Greedy thing," she said. "It's only been a couple of hours." She reached into the diaper bag and pulled out a bottle of formula.

"Why don't you breast-feed instead?" I said. "I can help you, if you have trouble."

"Well, okay," said Teresa. She pulled up her sweatshirt and undid her bra. Her round, full breasts fell against her still full belly. I handed the baby to her; hesitantly and a little awkwardly, she brought the baby's head to her right breast. As soon as the baby's lips touched Teresa's skin, her tiny mouth grabbed for the nipple and began to suck vigorously.

I laughed. "She seems to have the idea just fine," I said.

Teresa looked down at her. "Hurts when she first starts sucking," she said. "After that, it's not so bad."

"Are you getting custody of Ronald and Damian too?" I asked.

Teresa was silent for a few seconds before answering. "I don't know," she said. "My DSS worker, she wants me to. She keeps pushin' me, sayin' don't I want to get all my kids back. But I don't want to take on too much, y'know? If I take on too much I might want the drugs too bad, so's it won't feel so crazy. 'Sides, Ronald doesn't want to live with me. He don't even want to come visit me—he cries half the time he's with me, unless Damian's there. He likes bein' with Damian. Ronald, he wants to stay with his foster family—they's had him since he was a baby, they take real good care of him, and they been talkin' 'bout wantin' to adopt him. His daddy don't want him and that's good 'cause his daddy should never have no kid to take care of, he's a bad man. I'm his mama and I love him, but I been thinkin' that maybe he's better off where he is, y'know? I'm hopin' to stay clean, but I just don't know, y'know?" She looked up at me and her eyes were very sad.

"It sounds like whatever you do will be the right thing," I said, "because you're thinking about what's best for him."

"You think I'm bad, sayin' maybe I don't want my kid back?"

"Of course not. I think you love your child very much."

I reached out to touch her arm, but she moved in the chair; I couldn't tell if she was adjusting the baby or moving out of reach.

"And Damian?"

"I don't know 'bout Damian, either. Oh, I'll probably get him back. He knows me and we get on okay. But he's just gettin' so hard to control. He's only ten and he be out on the street all the time. He don't listen to me. He give me that smart-ass look and he be out the door fast as a wink. Even if I do get him back, I want him to spend time with his daddy. He listen to his daddy better than to me—his daddy beats him good if he don't."

I opened my mouth to say something about how it wasn't a good idea to beat children, but Teresa cut me off.

"I know, you're gonna say we shouldn't beat him. But hey, I got hit lots and I survived. And if it keeps him off the street, then it's fine by me, 'cause if he be on the streets too much he's gonna end up dead anyway."

This was hard to argue with, but I felt as if I should try. "What about after school programs, sports or something? What about calling the Y or the Boys and Girls Club? That might get him off the street and help his attitude too."

Teresa shrugged and looked past me. Clearly, that required more energy than she had at the moment. "Maybe the DSS worker could make the calls. You could talk to her."

Teresa shrugged again. I could see that she didn't see the need to search for a better solution when she had one that was adequate.

Lila came over to Teresa, pulling at her sleeve. "Mama, I'm hungry," she said.

"Just a minute," said Teresa. She looked at me. "You all done with the baby?" she asked. "I kept Lila home from school today 'cause I couldn't get her to school and get here on time, and I didn't have time to fix her breakfast."

"Yes," I said. I probably had other patients waiting at that point, too, I realized. "I'd like to see her again in a couple of weeks, to give her the second hepatitis shot. You can make the appointment on your way out."

Teresa took the baby off her breast and laid her on her lap while she refastened her bra and pulled her sweatshirt down. Then she picked Andrea up and brought her to the exam table to get her dressed. I stood up, picked up the baby's chart, and walked to the door.

"Mama, I'm *real* hungry," said Lila.

"I said just a minute," said Teresa sharply.

"We have graham crackers and juice," I said quickly. "I can take her to get some while you get the baby ready, if that's okay with you."

"Yeah, whatever," said Teresa without looking up.

I reached out my hand to Lila, who came right over to me. Her hand was soft and small in mine.

"I'll bring her right back," I said.

"Hmm," said Teresa.

As I walked down the hall with Lila, I reminded myself that sometimes progress is very slow. We must be careful not to expect too much or give up too soon.

Twenty-One

I wanted to talk with you about Teresa Dalton," I said.

"Teresa Dalton . . . oh, yeah," said the DSS worker, a young woman named Denise Reynolds. "I'm sorry—I just started at this office about a month ago, I'm still having trouble keeping the names straight. But I know who you're talking about. Is there a problem with Teresa? I thought things were going pretty well."

"Things are, actually. But I'm concerned about the plans to get her all the children back."

"Is there something going on I don't know about? I've only been out to see her twice, but she's been good with Lila and the baby, and the apartment has been clean and there's been food in the refrigerator. Her urine screens have been negative for any drugs. She's keeping all of her appointments, too, and she's done all the Medicaid and welfare paperwork. I haven't met Damian yet, but the worker who had the case before me said that she was good with him, too."

"So you want to give her custody of all of them?"

"Well . . ." Denise was clearly a little confused. "We think it's good for families to be reunited, and she's doing well. *Is* there something going on?"

"No. She's clean as far as I can tell, the baby's doing well, she's more involved and appropriate with Lila, and I think she does as well as anyone can with Damian. I just worry that it might be too much too soon to give her custody of them all."

"We're not rushing her," said Denise, sounding a bit defensive. "She is meeting all the requirements of her service plan. The case is coming up for review with my supervisor—gives me an opportunity to get her her kids back, since she's doing everything she needs to do to get them."

"Don't you think that getting her kids back should work around Teresa's schedule, not yours?"

As soon as I said this, I knew I wasn't being entirely fair. Any large bureaucracy like the child welfare system needs to have protocols and rules, or there will be chaos. The sheer volume of cases and workers brings with it an intrinsic limitation: the bureaucracy can't respond individually to each family's timetable. It needs, to some extent, to impose a timetable in order to ensure consistency and fairness. Not that the child welfare system is reliably consistent, or fair; people are not robots, and subjectivity, opinions, mistakes, and misconceptions always find their way in.

Smaller agencies can be more responsive. When those in charge can really know their employees, really know the cases and everything that is happening in them, there can be more room for flexibility. But having a bunch of smaller agencies doing the business of protecting children has its own set of limitations and problems because each agency could choose to be flexible in a different way. Accountability then becomes difficult, and the way different families are treated could come to depend on which agency the family ends up with rather than on agreed-upon standards. Neither, clearly, is a solution.

"I'm trying to work with Teresa, not against her," said Denise tersely.

"I know. I'm sorry. It's just that—"

"Besides," said Denise, cutting me off, "her kids need to know where they belong. They need security, instead of being in limbo like they are. They need some permanency."

"Don't you see that that's exactly what she's trying to give them?" I said. "She's trying to be sure that she can stay off drugs, because she can't keep them if she doesn't. She's trying to be sure that she can handle Damian, because she can't keep him if she can't handle him. And she's wondering if maybe she should just let Ronald keep the permanency he's got."

There was a silence before Denise said, "I guess we just see things differently than you do."

They are allowed to see things differently, of course. Who knows if the way I see things is right? Maybe neither of us is right. What would it take to be certain of being right? Certainly, it would take more information, and more time with Teresa, than either of us would ever have.

When there is an allegation of abuse or neglect made to DSS there is a period of investigation and assessment. During that visit, there are a number of visits in the home, with in-depth interviews of the parents and of the children. Other people are interviewed, too: teachers, doctors, neighbors, extended family, anyone who has contact with the family and might have information about what is going on. During that time, a relatively complete picture can be drawn. It may not be exactly correct—some interviewers are better at getting information than others, people lie, the people with the best information may be missed—but it's relatively complete.

After that, if the children are allowed to remain in the home, the worker usually visits only once a month. He or she may visit more often if there are particular concerns, but with the huge caseloads some of these workers carry, once a month is often the best they can do. Once a month, in an hour or so visit where the kids may be running around, making it hard to complete sentences let alone have a thorough conversation. Once a month to assess whether the kids are being fed and washed and cared for, to assess whether the parents are doing a good job.

Some situations are so bad, some parents are so strung out and damaged, that pulling things together for an hour a month isn't possible. But how hard is it, really, to run to the convenience store and pick up some food for the refrigerator, run the vacuum cleaner over the rug and put the trash in a closet, stick the kids in the bathtub and throw some water over them, and then smile a lot and be pleasant—for one hour a month? The incentive to lie and make things look good is very strong: if the parents don't, their children could be taken away. And even the best homes and families have at least one bad hour a month, when the house is a mess and there's no food around and the kids are a mess too and act so awful that you yell at them, loud, despite yourself. Who can tell anything definitively from an hour a month?

I see families less than an hour a month, usually. When children are under a year old they need to be seen about every couple of months, and if I get to spend half an hour with them, that's a lot. I see them more if they are sick in between, and obviously the more children there are, the more I see the family—but it's still not much.

Snapshots, that's all we get. We have to hope that the snapshots are reflective. But because they aren't always, we look for patterns, like the relative number of good visits versus worrisome ones, as well as school attendance and whether appointments with the doctor and dentist are kept. We look at tiny things within the snapshots, the small interactions that can be so telling: the way a child looks at his father, the way a mother does or doesn't reach for her child, the offhand remark that can be the most truthful thing said. We look for clues.

I have learned a lot from some DSS workers about the search for clues. I have spoken with some who are impressively watchful and insightful, who know how to pick out what's important and who quickly come to understand a family. They have the perfect mix of aptitude, training, and experience.

But many workers are young, inexperienced, with little training. They have only guidelines, protocols, and supervisors to guide them—supervisors who are supervising large numbers of cases and are physically incapable of spending a lot of time on each case.

The workers themselves may have over twenty cases. Turnover is high; I only know of one case that has had the same worker for four years. Every other case I know that has been open for more than a year has had more than one worker; one family has had four workers.

I don't blame the workers for leaving. It's a hard, depressing job going into people's homes and seeing what they do, trying so hard to make a difference, usually without much success—and the people the workers are trying to help often distrust and dislike them and sabotage their efforts. The pay is poor, the work relentless . . . I don't know that I could do it, either.

But a job that is difficult to start with becomes almost impossible with such turnover. Each time there is a new worker, he or she has to try to get to know the case, sifting through pages and pages of notes, if there is even time to do that. And he or she has to try to build a relationship with a family that may or may not have any interest in building a relationship with anyone. With each transition, precious time and ground can be lost. With each transition, a crack is created that children can slip through . . . and the chance of a good outcome lessens.

Not that there aren't good outcomes, because there are. Actually, the system seems to work best in the extremes.

I remember a sweet, blond-haired, green-eyed, rosy-cheeked baby girl named Jennifer who was a patient of mine. She was bright, walking and talking early, and coyly manipulative in a way that always made me laugh. Her mother had a long history of drug abuse, and had lost custody of another child, a boy, because she neglected him. She used drugs throughout the pregnancy with Jennifer, who was born prematurely and needed intensive care for almost a month after birth. The mother made it clear that she had no interest in giving up drugs, let alone in taking care of the baby, and disappeared from the hospital to the street.

Jennifer went home from the hospital in the care of Mrs. Navarro, a warm, funny woman who had been a foster parent for years. She stayed up night after night with the baby girl, who was irritable and a poor feeder because of her exposure to drugs. Mrs. Navarro patiently held her, fed her, and played with her, and Jennifer grew chubby, happy, and completely healthy. Mrs. Navarro had a big family of children, grandchildren, and foster children, all of whom loved the baby girl as a sister. There was no trace in Jennifer of the pain and desperation she had come from. She was saved.

Many children are saved, plucked from homes that were killing them physically or emotionally or both, and put into homes where they are cared for and loved and can blossom. In these situations, when the family is clearly abysmal, the system works.

It also works when the family is basically fine, but there are circumstances that have overstressed it. A 51A was filed by the police against one of the mothers in our practice when nobody came to pick up her children at school, for the third time. The school said, too, that the children had been missing a lot of school and frequently coming in hungry and dirty. When the DSS investigator went to the apartment he found that the mother was alone—the father had been jailed on weapons charges. She was very depressed by this, and overwhelmed by the care of her three children, one of whom had asthma that had been acting up much more than usual. She was also close to broke, as her husband had been the sole source of income. She had been relying on her sister to pick her children up on days when she was busy with the child who had asthma or just too depressed to get dressed and get out of the apartment to go to the school, which was a significant distance from the apartment and she didn't have a car. But although her sister would agree cheerfully to do it, she sometimes forgot.

The mother was warm and loving with the children, who responded to her equally warmly and lovingly. They were fed, but the mother admitted that sometimes she didn't have much to give them. They were a little late on their checkups, but it seemed to coincide with the father's leaving; prior to that the children had been up-to-date. The apartment was a mess, but more important, the entire building was infested with cockroaches and mice. This, I told the investigator, was probably the reason the younger child's asthma was acting up, as he was allergic to both.

The case was assigned to a worker, who got to work right away. She helped the mother sign up for food stamps, and helped her find a part-time job in a Laundromat while the kids were at school. She also helped her find a new apartment in a different public housing complex, which was a little smaller but had no cockroaches or mice—and it was closer to the school, so the mother could get there more easily and didn't have to rely as much on her sister.

Within a few months, there was a dramatic improvement. The mother said that she felt much more in control of her life, and no longer so sad and helpless. There was enough food at home, the children and the apartment were remarkably cleaner, and the younger child had fewer asthma attacks. The children's school attendance improved, and they were picked up every day. The family was better; the case was closed.

Where the child protection system is more likely to fall apart is in the situations in the middle, the ones that are neither severe or minor, the situations where it is all more vague. The alcoholic mother who admits that she continues to drink (and is frequently seen drunk) and has no intention of stopping, whose child is not physically abused and is clean and fed, but who misses a lot of school and doctor's appointments and has a mouth full of cavities waiting to be filled . . . the mother who uses drugs but keeps promising she'll stop, who moves in and out of drug rehab programs, who does a reasonably good job of parenting when she's clean (which she can sometimes be for months) and a lousy job of parenting when she's not.

There's another family that still haunts me. A mother brought in her four-year-old daughter, saying that the little girl had said that the mother's boyfriend had touched her "down there," pointing at her vaginal area. The mother said that the boyfriend had been alone with the child a few times while she ran out to the store, but that he denied ever having touched the little girl, and she said that she "kind of" believed him. "He does stuff," she said, "but not like that." When I asked her what kind of stuff he did do she said that in the past he had beaten her up. "But that was a long time ago," she said. There was no physical evidence of molestation when I examined the little girl, but that certainly didn't rule it out, and I filed a 51A. The worker helped the mother get a restraining order against the boyfriend, and arranged for the little girl to see a psychologist who specialized in children who had been abused. The girl had several sessions but never talked about any abuse, and the psychologist ended up saying that it was "inconclusive" whether she had been abused or not. With no "disclosure" from the child and no physical evidence, there were no charges brought against the boyfriend. The mother didn't renew the restraining order when it expired.

The DSS worker kept the case open, because she was concerned and a little uncomfortable with the situation. I was, too, especially when the mother began to seem depressed and started missing appointments for her daughter. She admitted that the boyfriend was back again, "here and there," but she insisted that she never left him alone with her daughter. She also insisted that he was not beating her, no matter how many times we gently asked. The DSS worker and I weren't sure that we believed her, but we didn't know what else to do.

All of these situations are potential time bombs. Not necessarily, of course; maybe everything will be fine for these families and the children will be unharmed. But maybe the alcoholic mother will pass out one afternoon and the little boy will wander out into the street and get killed—or maybe she'll kill him by driving drunk with him in the car. Anything could happen to the children of the drug-abusing mother during her periods of using, anything on the spectrum from not getting enough to eat to getting caught in the crossfire of those who sell the drugs. And who knows what is happening or could happen to the little girl who said once that she was touched, and her mother; maybe they are fine, maybe nothing happened—or maybe the girl is being molested and the mother is being beaten.

All the child protection system has in these cases, really, is the once-a-month visits, the hunches of the worker, the chance clue. All the child protection system can do is wait and see, and hope that there will be warning signs before something truly awful happens. Too often, there are not—or they are missed.

Even in the extremes, when the system works best, it's still not great. When Jennifer, the little girl cared for so beautifully by Mrs. Navarro, was a year and a half old her mother's sister stepped forward to claim her. Mrs. Navarro had been talking about adopting her, as the mother had never surfaced from the streets, but suddenly this woman appeared asking for custody, a woman who had never met Jennifer, and because she was family and Mrs. Navarro was just a foster mother, DSS granted her request. The woman had no children of her own, no experience raising children, and wasn't sure she would adopt Jennifer. Mrs. Navarro asked that she be able to visit with Jennifer after she went to live with her aunt, but after the first few visits, the aunt stopped being receptive to them, and the worker didn't push her as Mrs. Navarro had no particular legal right to visitation. It's two years later, and Mrs. Navarro has no idea where or how Jennifer is.

Some children stay with and are adopted by the first family they go to live with when they are put into foster care, but too often they move from family to family, possibly being separated from siblings, never really being sure how long they will stay and what will come next. Some children are never adopted, but move through the foster care system until adulthood, possibly from home to home, waiting for the convoluted, slow legal process to free them for adoption—if they are lucky enough to find adoptive parents. Yes, the children are almost definitely healthier and safer than they would have been with their biological parents. But what does it do to children to grow up that way? How many of them are left angry, or depressed, or both, with trouble trusting or having secure relationships, and with poor self-esteem? Too many, I fear.

And what about the mother whose children were being left stranded at school? She may very well never run into trouble again. But what if she loses the job at the Laundromat? Will she be able to find another job by herself? And does she have the skills to do anything else besides supervise washing machines and fold laundry, enough skills to get a job that might move her and her children out of poverty? What will happen when her husband gets out of jail? If she becomes overwhelmed, will she be able to meet the needs of her children—or will the family fall apart again?

Not that all this is the responsibility of DSS, because it isn't. But everything the worker did, as helpful as it was, was merely a Band-Aid. So we cross our fingers and hope that it was just a scrape that was covered with the Band-Aid, a scrape that will heal—and not something deeper and more dangerous.

The point is that the system doesn't *really* work. It can't police every household, let alone fix every household. And once a child has been neglected or abused, the damage done is real and can last a lifetime. If we really want to take care of children, we will need to stop more of them from having to enter the system in the first place. There will always be some neglected and abused children, no matter what we do; that's one of the sad realities of human nature, and because of this we will always need to have and generously support some sort of child protection agency. But a tremendous amount of neglect and abuse could be prevented.

It doesn't take a rocket scientist to come up with some of the major risk factors for abuse and neglect in this country, such as overwhelmed and isolated parents, substance abuse, poverty and its stresses, and domestic violence. There are no easy solutions for any of these, of course, but there are things that can be done. We could build and staff more community centers with parenting support groups, day care and after-school activities, outreach workers and other programs to strengthen families. We could create more drug treatment programs so that there are enough to meet the need. We could create more subsidized higher education and job training programs so that families could have a better chance of getting themselves out of poverty, and improve schools so that more children enter adulthood with marketable skills. We could increase the number and scope of domestic violence awareness and support programs, so that help is always close by.

We do some of this, of course. But we don't do enough; as a country, we have tremendous inertia. Some politicians say that to do all this would create a Big Government, like an Orwellian Big Brother, that would go inside people's homes and invade their privacy—and a Big Government that would have too many regulations, stifle individual initiatives, and cost a lot of money.

The only argument that absolutely rings true is that it would cost a lot of money. We would have to spend much more on social programs and education than we are currently spending, and many people say that we don't have enough money to do this. I don't think that's true; I think that we have enough money in this country to take care of our people. It would mean building fewer bombers, granting fewer government subsidies, and it would mean that some of our multimillionaires and corporations would have to give up a million or two . . . but the money is there.

There is a family in my practice that DSS has been supporting very well for the past two years, when it became clear that a mother with a long history of drug abuse (and emotional trauma preceding that) could not take care of her newborn daughter and two-year-old son. She admitted it herself, as she left to go to the drug treatment program, where she never showed up. The children were put in the custody of the newborn's father, a soft-spoken, pleasant man in his late fifties.

Mr. Ramos lived alone. He had stopped working a few years before after a back injury, and lived off his disability check. He had grown children, but he had never actually participated in raising them, and it was obvious he was going to need help with taking care of two small children. Within a couple of weeks, the worker realized that he was going to need a lot of help, because not only had he no experience, but he couldn't read and had a learning disability that made learning new tasks very difficult for him. Although he had emigrated to the United States from Puerto Rico more than twenty-five years before, his English was still poor.

DSS found a day care program that did intensive parenting teaching and support. A couple of days a week, Mr. Ramos stayed at the day care with the children. He learned how to bathe them and dress them, and how to diaper the baby. He learned what he should feed them, and how best to wash the baby's bottles. He learned how to play with them. "You can talk to the baby," the day care teacher told him. "But she doesn't talk back," he said, genuinely confused. He learned how to organize his day at home, how to juggle caring for the children, doing errands, cooking, and doing laundry.

I enrolled the children in Early Intervention, a program for children at risk for developmental problems, and they sent someone to work with the children and Mr. Ramos either at home or at the day care. The worker from Early Intervention did developmental stimulation with the baby, and taught Mr. Ramos ways he could do it himself—which was again basically teaching him how to play with them. The DSS worker arranged for a Parent Aide to go to his house to reinforce what he was learning and to be a necessary spare pair of hands.

Mr. Ramos has made remarkable progress. The first time I saw them all after the children went to live with him, the baby had a bald spot at the back of her head from sitting in her baby chair at home all day doing nothing but watching television with him. She stared at me quietly from her stroller with a dirty face and big eyes. The little boy barely spoke, and sat curled up in the chair as if he wanted to disappear. Now when they come to the clinic they fill the exam room with laughter and motion. The baby is two years old and flourishing. She loves to climb all over Mr. Ramos, who smiles and tosses her in the air and then hugs her. The little boy is still shy but he no longer curls up in the chair; he plays with his sister and Mr. Ramos, and tells me in his small, clear voice about his favorite toys. He has grown from waifish to healthy and strong.

There is still work to be done, though. Mr. Ramos still can't read; I have to draw pictures whenever the children need medication and even with that they don't always get the medicine correctly. His English has improved, but only slightly. He misses appointments frequently. Every time I tell him anything, I have to call the day care staff and tell them too, so that with repetition and reminding it may sink in. He admits that weekends get hard, especially when the Parent Aide can't come over—he finds himself overwhelmed by the competing needs of the children. When he talks about this it is obvious that the services DSS has provided are the glue holding the family together; without them, things fall apart.

Thankfully, DSS has kept the case open, even though there is really isn't an official reason; there is no abuse or neglect, and since Mr. Ramos adopted the little boy both children are legally his and not foster children. But before long, DSS will have to close it; there are, after all, not enough resources to go around and there are families in much worse shape than this one. Hopefully, Mr. Ramos will have made more progress by the time the case is closed, but it's possible he won't have, and this thought terrifies me.

DSS isn't the only way to hold this family together, I think as I draw another picture of a medication bottle with a clock next to it so that Mr. Ramos knows what time to give his daughter the antibiotic for her ear infection. I can keep a special eye on this family, and make sure that they have a caseworker to coordinate appointments and help Mr. Ramos with insurance and bills and other difficult details of life. His friends and neighbors, or his grown children, could do things like help him read instructions, help him shop and cook, watch the little boy while Mr. Ramos gives the little girl her bath, or help the children with their homework when they get to be school age. There are hundreds of simple ways that the people whose lives touch Mr. Ramos's could help him take care of his children.

There are hundreds of simple ways that all of us can help people take care of their children, and in doing so possibly prevent abuse and neglect. Every day, we are presented with opportunities: we could let a mother with a crying child go ahead of us in line, cook a meal for a family when one of the parents is sick, befriend the lonely new family on the block, offer to baby-sit . . . and yet, somehow, this doesn't happen anywhere near as much as it should. Too often, we live tightly inside insular little worlds, rarely reaching out. This kind of inertia is as much a part of the problem as, and is probably the root of, our political inertia.

We are going to have to come out of our little worlds. We are going to have to reach out. We are going to have to get past our inertia, both personal and political. The lives of too many children are at stake.

Twenty-Two

*L*uz had been growing more and more worried.

Most of it was Kevin. I was getting worried, too; he was having more trouble with the sickle-cell anemia than usual for his age. The frequent hospitalizations for fevers were continuing. Between visits, he was getting pain in his hands and feet from the sickling of the red cells in his blood, pain bad enough to require codeine. He wasn't eating very well, probably because of the fevers and the pain, so his weight gain was poor. Luz did everything we told her to: she gave him high-calorie foods, she made sure he drank enough so that he wouldn't get dehydrated and have even more pain, and she gave him each medication exactly as directed. But nothing made much difference; sickle-cell anemia can be an independent and powerful disease.

I could tell that Luz was worried about more than Kevin, though; even on days when he was doing well the frown did not lift from her face. Finally, one day when I asked her yet again what else was wrong, she asked me what I knew about the laws regarding custody of children.

I asked her why. She said that Ricardo had been saying that he was going to get her declared an unfit mother and take Kevin away from her.

I took a deep breath. Luz had not said anything about Ricardo for two or three months. Each time I had asked about him, her face had gone blank and she had shrugged and said everything was fine. When I had asked questions about her safety she had repeated that everything was fine and then quickly and firmly changed the subject.

"*Pero Ud. es una madre muy buena,*" I said—you're a very good mother. I said that I and lots of other people would testify to that. And if she got the restraining order, not only might it keep her safer but it would help show that Ricardo shouldn't have custody of Kevin.

She frowned. She hesitated for a moment, and then said that he was also threatening to have her deported.

"*¿Para tomar a Kevin?*" I asked—to get Kevin?

She shrugged. "*De veras, yo no creo que realmente quiere cuidar a Kevin. Es a mí a quien quiere hacer daño.*" She didn't think he really wanted to take care of Kevin. She thought he just wanted to hurt her.

I asked how he could get her deported, since she had all the appropriate visas and paperwork to be here. She said she didn't know—probably by making up some sort of lie about her. He was capable of almost anything. She asked if I knew how she could get her citizenship faster—did Kevin's illness make any difference?

Kevin was a citizen because he was born here, but perhaps the case could be made that he needed to be with his mother for his best emotional and physical health, and he needed to be in the United States rather than the Dominican Republic because his sickle-cell disease was particularly bad and here there was better access to good health care—so it would be best for him if his mother were a citizen. I said that she needed to talk to a lawyer about both the custody and the immigration issues. She said that she had no money; I said that she could get free legal advice at Greater Boston Legal Services. I offered to go with her, to trans-late. I could have sent her with the caseworker, but I figured that I would be better able to explain Kevin's medical needs.

We arranged to meet at the clinic a few days later, on one of my days off. I asked my mother-in-law to baby-sit for Michaela and Zachary, as Mark was working all day into the evening. Legal Ser-vices started seeing people at one, on a first-come first-serve basis, so I asked Luz to be at the clinic at around twelve-thirty to allow us time to drive there and find parking. She agreed, and smiled. She looked more hopeful than I had seen her in a while.

The day came, a bitterly cold November Wednesday. She was late. She rushed in to the lobby with Kevin on her hip, neither of them dressed warmly enough against the cold wind. Luz wore a sweater and skirt that were pretty but wrinkled and not very clean, and her pantyhose had a long, wide run down one leg. Her hair, instead of being carefully combed back and wound into a knot, was pulled back messily and tied with a rubber band.

I opened my mouth to ask if she was okay, and Kevin started to whine. Luz bounced him on her hip, a little desperately; he didn't stop. I wasn't going to be able to talk to her, I could see, so I motioned her to the car.

Luz wanted to hold Kevin in her lap in the front seat. I insisted that he be strapped into Zachary's car seat in the back; it was much safer, I explained. She acquiesced, but as I leaned past her to adjust the straps, I could see that she was holding back tears.

Kevin quieted once the car started moving; the car seat was clearly a new experience for him, and I could tell that he liked being high up enough to see out the windows. Luz was quiet, staring ahead. When we stopped at the intersection at South Huntington she reached into her purse, pulled out a business card, and handed it to me.

"*Esta persona quiere que Ud. la llame,*" she said—this person wants you to call her.

I looked down at the card. Sergeant Eileen McDougall, it said. Sexual Assault Unit.

I pulled the car over to the side of the road and turned off the engine. Trying to keep calm, I asked her what happened. "*¿Qué pasó?*"

In an equally calm voice Luz told me that Ricardo had raped her.

I undid my seat belt, reached over, and gave her a hug. All of a sudden her tears began to flow, and with them came tumbling out words, disjointed, filling out the story. Ricardo had broken the window of her back door at dawn to get in; he surprised her in bed. He pulled her from there, beat her, and raped her.

As she spoke, I suddenly noticed bruises along her neck and the side of her face that she had tried to cover with makeup.

She screamed, she told me. The neighbors must have heard her, because somebody called the police who came in time to catch Ricardo as he was leaving the apartment. They took him away somewhere, she said, and then took her to Boston City Hospital, where lots of people talked to her and they took pictures and "did all those tests." It took a long time, she said, which was why she was late.

"Tuve que dejar a Kevin con mis vecinos. Todo el tiempo que yo estuve en el hospital yo me preocupé mucho por él, porque no los concía." She had to leave Kevin with the neighbors, and while she was at the hospital she was very worried about him, because he didn't know the neighbors. Her voice was a little breathless through her tears.

I asked her why she had come to meet me. We didn't need to go to Legal Services that day; we could go some other time. Didn't she want to go home?

She shook her head. She didn't want to go home. Her landlord might be fixing the window. She would need to clean up. She couldn't go there, not now.

I asked if there was a friend or family member she wanted to call or go see. I offered to drive her anywhere she wanted to go.

She shook her head again. She had one friend, she said, but she was in New York City visiting relatives for a few days. Her sister was at work. Besides, Luz said, her sister would be angry—angry at Ricardo, and angry at Luz for not listening to her when she said that Ricardo was a bad man. She wasn't ready to see her, not yet.

Her voice gathered strength. *"Quiero ver al abogado,"* she said clearly—I want to see the lawyer. She said that Ricardo would be very angry to be in jail, and he would want to hurt her—and he might tell lies about her or get his brother to tell lies about her to get her deported or get Kevin taken away. She wanted to see the lawyer, so that she could be ready.

I said that we could talk to the lawyer about what happened. She shook her head vigorously. No, she said, the police had already talked to her about it. She wasn't going to talk about it again. She only wanted to talk about her citizenship and keeping custody of Kevin.

I started up the car. We drove to downtown Boston in silence, found a metered parking spot on the street, and went into the lobby of Greater Boston Legal Services. It was nearly two o'clock, and there were a number of people waiting. The secretary said that it would probably be at least an hour before we were seen. Luz and I sat down in the last two chairs remaining in the waiting room. Kevin started to whine again; Luz pulled out a half-empty bottle from her purse and gave it to Kevin, who drained it quickly and started to cry.

"*¿Ha comido hoy?*" I said—has he eaten today?

Luz shook her head.

"*¿Has comido hoy?*"—have you eaten today?

She shook her head again.

I told her I'd be right back, and went in search of food. The only place I could find was a narrow, dark, dusty deli a few doors down that sold sandwiches and not much else. I stared at the menu, having no idea what Luz and Kevin would like; when the man behind the counter started to get annoyed with me I ordered a cheese sandwich and a turkey sandwich. I bought containers of milk and juice, too, and a Coke.

I went back to Legal Services and gave the sandwiches and drinks to Luz. She unwrapped the white waxed paper packages a little uncertainly. She put Kevin on the floor in front of her, separated the cheese sandwich into bread and cheese and tore them into small pieces, and laid it all down in front of him on the waxed paper. He began to grab handfuls of bread and cheese and shove them into his mouth. She poured the milk into his empty bottle, screwed the nipple back on, and handed that to him; he took the bottle and sucked on it vigorously in between handfuls of food.

She opened the Coke for herself and took a few long sips, staring straight ahead, before picking up the sandwich and beginning to eat. She took big bites, obviously hungry, but she chewed and swallowed awkwardly, as if it were a tremendous effort.

I watched the two of them sit and eat, oblivious to everything around them, softly radiating vulnerability and pain.

I touched Luz on the shoulder; she looked at me as if she'd nearly forgotten I was there. I asked her if she'd been able to take a long shower or bath yet that day.

She shook her head. She didn't have time, she told me. She had just taken a quick shower when she was getting ready to meet me. When she got home she would try to get Kevin to sleep so that she could take a long shower.

I imagined her going home to the apartment where she had been beaten and raped hours earlier. Maybe the window would be fixed, but maybe the gaping hole and the scattered glass would still be there and she would have to clean it up and cover the hole herself. I imagined her trying to feed, bathe, and dress Kevin by herself and then rock him to sleep in the apartment whose walls probably still echoed with her screams.

"*¿Quieres pasar la noche en mi casa?*" The image was too much for me; I invited her home for the night. I had a couch that pulled out into a bed, I told her, and as Kevin and Zachary were the same age, I had clothes and diapers that would fit Kevin. I could watch him, and she could shower or rest or do whatever she wanted. She didn't have to, of course—I would be happy to bring her back to her apartment—but would she like to come home with me?

She looked straight at me. A quiet, small smile came into her eyes, and she nodded.

She went back to eating her sandwich, and I felt something like panic grip me. Had I just done something I wasn't supposed to do? Had I just crossed one of those lines you should never cross?

When I was in medical school the older physicians who taught us spoke frequently about maintaining a certain "distance" from patients. The main reason seemed to be that if we became too close emotionally to a patient, it could impair our judgment as we made medical decisions for and about them. Another reason, somewhat less emphasized, was that we might seek to gain something from the relationship with the patient and thereby exploit him or her, inappropriately using our position of power; an example given was of a psychiatrist seducing a depressed and vulnerable patient.

All of that seemed to make good sense. But it was never entirely clear to me just what the definition of "distance" was, or how it was to be created. It felt odd to be asking the terribly personal questions we were taught to ask and then offering nothing of ourselves that was personal in return. But the point wasn't to build a relationship with the patient; it was to gather information and make good medical decisions.

Or was it? We *were* supposed to be building a relationship with the patient, so that they would trust us, listen, tell us what we needed to know, and follow instructions. Yet the relationship was incredibly artificial and one-sided, with the physician holding the authority, with no mandate to share much of anything. And it seemed that too often physicians used "therapeutic distance" as an excuse to be brief, brusque—even unkind. Instead of something to protect the patient, it became something to protect the physician— from the emotionally difficult task of being involved in another person's life.

It didn't have to be that way, I was certain. If we were cautious, respectful, and honest—especially with ourselves—we could be friends with our patients. It would be harder than being distant and whisking in and out of the exam room, but it could be done without being exploitative or compromising our judgment, and I felt sure it would lead to better care for patients. Doctors know medicine, but they don't know what it is to be the particular patient. They can't know all patients' fears or habits or beliefs, which are intrinsic to their health, or the details of their lives that interfere with the best of medical plans—this is expertise that only the patient holds. If we are partners with patients, there is a sharing of expertise, which leads to better medical outcomes as well as better communication and trust. The relationship becomes more normal, more human, more kind.

And some situations, I thought, demanded that we react first as people and second as doctors. I was sitting with a woman who had just been beaten and raped, who was alone with a small child to take care of. I had something to offer that would help, something as simple as sharing my home for a night, and I couldn't live with myself if I didn't offer it.

We finally saw the lawyer, or rather the law student, who was very nice. Luz chose only to ask questions about citizenship, not about custody issues, and she didn't mention anything about the rape. I respected her decision, and did not add anything as I translated. The law student clearly and pleasantly discussed options and procedures; I translated and Luz nodded but I don't think she was really listening. We thanked him and left.

My mother-in-law greeted us warmly when we arrived home; she'd cleaned up the house, for which I was grateful. As she was leaving, she told me to call if I needed any help or anything from the store. Michaela and Zachary were as usual happy to have guests. Michaela, who was nearly three and quite the little hostess, immediately started bringing toys to Kevin, who sat down in the middle of the living room floor and stared with wonderment at the growing pile. Zachary, who was fifteen months old, sat near him and babbled unintelligibly, stopping every once in a while to grab a favorite toy out of the pile.

I got a big soft sweatshirt, some knit pants that had shrunk and so were too short for me, and some warm wool socks and brought them to Luz. I showed her the bathroom and got her a clean towel from the closet. I told her to take as long as she wanted. She was in there for more than half an hour, the steam of a very hot shower seeping out around the door and into the hall.

When Luz came out, her skin pink and her hair neatly combed, she said that she wanted to cook our dinner. I said that I would be happy to cook, that she should just rest, but she insisted; it seemed so important to her that I gave in. We hunted together through the cabinets and the refrigerator; she pulled out some white rice, some canned kidney beans, a tomato, an onion, some cloves of garlic, and various spices and made a wonderfully fragrant dish of rice and beans. We sat with the children at the little kitchen table; all three of them ate ravenously, and laughed with and at each other. Luz and I smiled at them, played with them, helped them with their food. The light from the hanging lamp over the table glowed, and mixed with the laughter, made a circle of warmth.

When we had finished Luz stood up to clear the table; as she took the plates to the sink, her hands shook ever so slightly, and her steps were slow, as if suddenly it was hard for her to lift her feet from the floor. I took the plates from her and brought her into the living room. I motioned for her to lie down on the couch, which she did; I covered her with the soft cotton throw. I brought her a glass of white wine; she took it from me and sipped it slowly. I asked her if she wanted the lights on or off; off, she said.

I went back to the kitchen and did the dishes and otherwise cleaned up. The children played underfoot, hiding under the table, playing with mixing bowls and wooden spoons. Michaela had a sturdy plastic play kitchenette with a pretend stove and sink and a cabinet underneath; Kevin climbed into the cabinet and played peek-a-boo with Michaela and Zachary, who found this uproariously funny.

When I'd finished cleaning up I brought them into the bathroom. I filled the tub with hot water and bubble bath and put all three of them in together. Kevin seemed a little unsure, and looked around for Luz, but soon the bubbles and the bath toys distracted him and he played happily with Michaela and Zachary. I washed his thick dark hair and cleaned his dark, smooth skin with a washcloth. Although I'd known he was thin from his growth chart, it was startling to see how small and frail he looked next to my robust children. I took him out first, dried him with a fluffy towel and put on a clean diaper and a pair of warm blue pajamas that I'd pulled out of Zachary's drawer.

It felt good to do the simple tasks of bathing and dressing him. So many times when I saw children at the clinic I would reach for the bottles to feed them when they were hungry, or I would start to change their diapers when they were wet, or I would want to comfort them when they cried, but their mothers swooped in and did it first. I would realize yet again that it wasn't officially my job as a pediatrician to do those tasks, that those were my jobs as a mother. It seemed odd, and unnatural, that I should be expected to be either a doctor or a mother but not both. As I did the snaps under Kevin's chin, I was glad to be able to take care of a child in every way I knew how.

By the time Mark came home from work all three children were in their pajamas and ready for bed. He played with them all, tossing Kevin into the air just as he did with Michaela and Zachary, much to Kevin's delight. Luz sat up on the couch and talked with Mark and me, with me acting as translator. We talked about the children, the house, the dog (whom I had left tied up outside), the clinic. Luz laughed as she talked; watching her, Kevin's face lit up. We did not talk about the rape. There would be time for that later.

Mark helped me pull the couch out into a bed and put on flannel sheets and some blankets. I asked Luz if she wanted me to set up the portable crib, but she said no. She wanted Kevin with her.

In the morning we had a quick breakfast before getting back into the car to drive to Boston. Luz agreed to keep the pants, as they were too small for me, and the socks, as I convinced her that I had plenty and her pantyhose were no longer wearable. We decided that Kevin should wear Zachary's pajamas under his clothes, as it was cold. She could give them back to me some other time, I told her, hoping she wouldn't.

When we were in the car I asked her what would happen next.

"*No sé,*" she said, staring out at the highway—I don't know.

I would call the sergeant, I told her. I would find out what would happen next. I would talk to the caseworker when I got to the clinic. We would help her through it all.

Luz nodded. I don't know if she was listening. Her eyes didn't move from the highway. The gray sky melded at the horizon with the gray of the pavement.

I asked her how to get to her apartment. She shook her head and told me to go to the clinic. Her sister lived near there, close enough to walk. It was time to tell her what had happened, she said. She would see if she could stay with her for a while.

Soon we were there and she was lifting sleepy Kevin from the car seat and putting him onto her hip. He lay his head on her shoulder; she swung her purse over the other shoulder and turned to me.

"*Gracias,*" she said.

"*De nada,*" I said—you're welcome.

Luz turned and walked up Bickford Street toward Centre Street. I stood by my car, watching her go. The wind blew hard against her; she pulled Kevin closer, ducked her head down, and leaned forward, making her steps longer.

As I stood there watching her, I felt helpless against her pain, against the awful things that had happened to her. I wished that there was more that I could do; instead of just sharing my home, I wished that I could wipe away the badness, make her world safe, take away her son's disease. But such things are impossible. We are limited to doing the best we can.

Twenty-Three

When the summer of 1994 arrived I'd had three years of experience in both motherhood and practicing pediatrics at Martha Eliot. While I didn't exactly feel adept at either, that summer was something of a turning point for me. Nothing in particular happened—perhaps it was just the passage of time—but I found myself less awkward at both motherhood and pediatrics, more comfortable with and certain of both.

Zachary turned two that summer, talkative and so affectionate and endearing that he got the nickname Bug, short for Lovebug. Michaela was three and a half; her tantrums had faded into a willfullness that alternately exasperated me and made me laugh. She was finally out of diapers, after a long struggle, and very excited about the nursery school she was going to attend in the fall. I no longer felt overwhelmed by the tasks of two children. I had found routines and tricks that worked, and some confidence along the way too. Which isn't to say that there weren't new challenges and frustrations daily, but by that summer I had accepted them; I had accepted the fact that parenthood is a continually humbling experience.

It was much the same with practicing pediatrics at Martha Eliot; I had acknowledged and accepted that as a continually humbling experience as well. But by the summer of 1994 I knew the routines and flow of the clinic, I had grown used to hearing and speaking Spanish, and I was accustomed to the logistics and the limitations of inner-city primary care. I'd come to know the families better too: their personalities, their weaknesses, their strengths—and this made being their doctor much easier. I knew better what to expect from them, and what to do to help them.

I saw Carlos Molina one day that July for a bad scrape on his knee; Señora Gonzalez thought it might need stitches, but luckily it didn't. She had already scrubbed it well at home, so there was not much for me to do but pronounce it not in need of stitches and put on a bandage. As I did, Carlos told me how it happened: he fell off his new bike, he said. He was racing the boy who lived across the street. There was a bump in the road, and the bike skidded, but he won the race. His face beamed with pride.

New bike? I wondered how the Gonzalez family could afford that. Señora Gonzalez smiled. It was her son's old one, she said. They'd dragged it out of the basement, mended and oiled it, and painted it shiny red.

"It's great," said Carlos. "It's the best thing I ever had." I'd never seen him so happy. He jumped off the table when I finished bandaging, full of confidence and strength.

When he was out in the waiting room Señora Gonzalez told me in a hushed voice that the psychologist was saying it was time to move Daisy to a specialized foster home because she was still doing dangerous things and the psychologist was concerned for her safety and the safety of everyone in the house.

Señora Gonzalez was clearly upset by this, to the point of tears. She was doing her best to give Daisy lots of love, she said, but it wasn't stopping Daisy from being so angry and mean and setting the fires.

Maybe she'll go away for a while, get some intensive help, I said, and then come back to you happy and well. Señora Gonzalez shrugged; she didn't look particularly hopeful that this would happen. To be honest, I wasn't either. There was something in Daisy's eyes that made me feel like the damage ran deep.

Kevin was hospitalized three times that summer, for fever and pain. Ricardo was in jail awaiting his trial; he couldn't make bail, for which I was very thankful. The District Attorney's office was hounding Luz, wanting to be sure she was willing to testify. She said that she would. She said this resolutely, but there was a soft tremor in her voice, and sometimes I thought that she might just disappear.

I saw Teresa that summer too, when she came in for Andrea's physical and shots. She was still drug-free. Breast-feeding didn't work out, but Andrea was growing and full of smiles. Lila looked good, too, and the interactions between her and Teresa were warmer. DSS decided to delay plans to give Teresa custody of Damian and Ronald. It had nothing to do with my phone call, the DSS worker was careful to tell me. It was because Teresa had a new-born baby, and they were going to give her some time to adjust.

I didn't see Joan that summer. Timothy was overdue for a physical, and I called Joan's mother's house several times. She was vague, saying she would give Joan the message. I wondered if maybe she didn't know where Joan was, either.

I figured that Joan was probably using drugs again. But maybe she wasn't. Or if she was, I thought, maybe tomorrow something would happen that would change her world just enough to give her the will to try to stop—that little bit of luck, like getting off the waiting list for an apartment, or that something that one of her children said or did that was jarring and undeniable. If not tomorrow, maybe it would be the next day, or the one after that. There are so many tomorrows, and so many chances.

Lives can never truly be predicted; they are much more elusive than that. They can change on a dime. The possibilities are endless, both good and bad, and the story is never completely written until you die.

I think that's a lot of what gets me through the days at Martha Eliot: believing in people's possibilities. Badness happens—but there is always a reason to hope.

I still feel in between worlds, or countries, between where and how I grew up and where and how I work. That hadn't changed by the summer of 1994 and hasn't changed in the years since. It never will change, because I can't change my past. I will never completely know what it is to grow up in the inner city. But being in between bothers me less now; that I fit in perfectly anywhere doesn't matter so much anymore. My life has become defined more by the faces and moments that fill it than by any other parameter—and this, I have found, is more than enough. I love doing inner-city primary care, and I will probably do it for the rest of my career.

I have a friend from residency who went to work in a private practice in a wealthy suburb of Boston. One day we compared the kind of conversations we had with the families in our respective practices. She is able to take it for granted that the families she sees have a safe place to live and the money to buy food and medicine, so her conversations tend to be about specific medical issues or about behavior and child-rearing concerns. Certainly she asks personal questions if she senses that there is something wrong, but in general, the conversations are fairly superficial. I, on the other hand, can take nothing for granted. I have to ask a lot of questions that in my friend's practice would be considered prying. The conversations that grow from my questions are about everything and anything. We talk about the details of families' living situations, including the conditions of the walls and the names, ages, and sleeping locations of everyone in the household. We talk about exactly what they eat, and how much money they have to spend each month as I try to figure out what medications I can prescribe. We talk about their neighborhoods, and what kind of violence their children see and how they keep the children safe. The single mothers and I talk about the patterns and frustrations of their days, how they cope, how they might better fight against the challenges of raising children on their own in the inner city. With the teenage mothers, I talk about absolutely everything, from diapering to their

own education, for I can't take it for granted that they know anything at all about parenting—and I don't want them to lose their
chance at a future.

And then there are the unexpected bits of information. *"Otra cosa,
doctora"*—one more thing, Doctor—the mothers or fathers or aunts
say as they are just about to leave. Was it normal, one mother asked,
that since visiting with an older male cousin her six-year-old daughter was talking graphically about sex? Another mother timidly told
us as she was headed out the door that her husband was halluci-
nating. A father told me that his wife was using cocaine and he didn't
know what to do. I am sure that this happens in suburban practices,
too, but what runs under the surface of my patients' lives can be
more desperate and more dangerous.

My friend is undeniably part of her patients' lives. But it is different for me. By necessity, I am drawn in deeper—and I am grateful for this.

I love the practice of medicine. I love the tricky, complicated
process of making a diagnosis, a process that relies equally on
knowledge and instinct. In primary care it is especially challenging, because the primary care physician is the front line, the one
who sees a hundred stomachaches and has to pick out the appen-
dicitis or the tumor from the ninety-eight with a virus. I love
watching symptoms and illnesses improve with the right medication—the wheezing child who after some nebulized albuterol no
longer has trouble breathing, the listless toddler burning with
fever who is running happily down the hall after ibuprofen, the
swollen, painful skin infection cured with antibiotics. But more
than any of this, I love being witness to the richness of human
experience.

I suppose that I could be accused of voyeurism, for indeed, I do
like watching other people's lives. But that's because I've always
thought that people are the best part of life, the only part that is
truly worthwhile and interesting. Everything else—careers, poli-

tics, the arts, sports, everything—is overlay and would not exist without the common denominator of people.

There is much about human nature that is unappealing and disappointing, of course. There is cruelty and selfishness. People lie, steal, and murder. But there is so much, and I believe so much more, that is great. People have the capacity for tremendous love, strength, and courage. They have the ability to rise to occasions and challenges, and to even sometimes make a miracle.

I get to see this every day at Martha Eliot. For most of the families who come to see us there, life is a constant struggle. There is little buffer between them and badness: poverty, hunger, homelessness, violence. Just the fact of making it through each day is an achievement of which to be proud. That most of them make it through the days safe, and happy, and that many manage to stay hopeful, represents incredible resilience, determination, and faith. Day after day, I am inspired. And day after day, I am given chance after chance to make a friend and make a difference, even if the differences I make are very small. This is the best part of my job: it connects my life to many others.

Working at Martha Eliot, I have seen clearly just how much people need each other. It isn't just about survival; it's also about sustenance, the sustenance of heart and mind.

It makes us happy to be successful, of course. It makes us happy to have enough money to be able to buy lots of nice things, and to have a nice place to live. It makes us happy to get a good job, and to be promoted. It makes us happy to create art, music, literature, or simply do something well. It makes us happy to feel powerful.

But none of that compares to how it makes us feel to fall in love, or stay in love for years and years. None of it compares to how it feels to hold our children, or how it feels to be held close ourselves when we are filled with joy or pain. None of it compares to our gratitude for the outstretched hand when we need it, or what we feel in our hearts when we know we have truly helped or made someone happy. It is the connections between us that really make living worthwhile.

We know this well as children, when nothing matters more than our parents and our brothers and sisters and our friends. We know it as we grow old and away from our jobs and our distractions, suddenly finding ourselves with time on our hands; we find ourselves looking for friends and wishing for more time with our grown children and our grandchildren, fighting off loneliness. But in between, we too often forget.

It's easy to forget when we get busy with earning a living and keeping up with the details of life. And except for the occasional Hallmark movie or Christmas special, the importance of the connections between people doesn't get much airtime. Our society is deeply steeped in the capitalist mythology that each person should be able to stand on his own, should be able to be independent and pull himself up by his bootstraps, that success is defined by how much he has at the end. This mythology has made some millionaires, but it has made countless others lonely, discouraged, hungry, and poor.

We are our brothers' keepers. We need to be; it's that simple. For the survival of each one of us, and for humans as a species and Earth as a planet, depends on each other. Sooner or later we are going to have to realize this, and later may just be too late. Already, far too many people are desperate and dying—and it is well within our ability as a society to do something to stop it.

It would mean making a decision to make the welfare of all of our people our highest priority. Not just a priority, but the highest priority—higher than wealth or power. We would have to trust that if our people were well it would benefit everyone.

I'm not suggesting that the government pay everyone's bills, or that we all need to be Mother Teresas. The government would need to pay a few more bills, but its more important task would be reorganizing and remodeling its spending and programs to better support communities, education, and families. And the task of each one of us would be to share more of what we have. Those who have a lot of money would need to give some away, but we all have something we can share: our skills, our time, our friendship. Doctors, lawyers, and other professionals could work some portion of their time in underserved communities, but it can also be more simple: anything from volunteering in public schools, to helping a neighbor with home repairs, visiting elderly shut-ins, being a mentor to a teenager . . . the possibilities are endless, and it doesn't have to be a lot of work. If enough people do a little, the effect can be huge.

Lots of people are helping already. I meet them every day, and read about them in the newspaper; knowing that they exist keeps me hopeful. If there could just be more like them, if helping could become so common that it becomes ordinary, then not only would more people be helped but the politicians would take their cue from their constituents and guide the government toward helping more, too.

We also need to listen carefully to those we are trying to help. We cannot assume that we know what is best, or that we understand what it is to be anyone else but ourselves. Each life has reasons and boundaries that must be respected, and the best solutions for problems may not be obvious. We need to ask people for their ideas, taking the people and their needs on their own terms, in their own homes and neighborhoods. We need to treat people not as statistics or categories, but as brothers.

I close my eyes now and see the young men as they go off to work or stand against the buildings. I see them coming in with the women and smiling as I compliment their babies, holding the babies with pride. I see the women with their children in the waiting room or in the exam rooms breast-feeding, or walking along the streets with the strollers and the diaper bags; I see their faces as they light up or melt into tears, I hear their voices as they tell me about their babies and their lives. I see them all in my mind and I know absolutely that we are all so much more alike than we are different. Our needs, our desires, and our dreams are so very much the same—if not in their specifics, at least in their themes. We all need food, shelter, clothes, and money. We all want to be loved. We all want to be given a chance. And we all have the same right to all this as anyone else.

When I look into the eyes of the children I see at the clinic, when I play with them and plead with them, in their faces I see the faces of my children. As they talk with me and sing for me, I hear the voices of my children. And when they are in my arms—when I scoop up the newborns to examine them, or help the older children onto the exam table, or lift a toddler onto my hip to hold while his mother chases another child—they feel like my children and I know in my heart that they *are* my children. They are everyone's children, for they are everyone's future.

It is the early morning of their lives; anything, really, is still possible. They deserve a chance. I hope that we can give them one.

About the Author

Claire McCarthy is an Ivy League–educated doctor, author, wife, and mother. After a three-year residency at Children's Hospital of Boston, McCarthy went to work as a primary-care pediatrician at the Martha Eliot Health Center located in the Bromley-Heath Housing Development in Jamaica Plain, a community of Boston. McCarthy chronicled her experiences as a medical student and resident in a series of vignettes which were first published in *The Boston Globe* and later published in book form as *Learning How the Heart Beats* (Viking, 1995). McCarthy is currently a regular columnist for *Sesame Street Parents* magazine. She lives in Melrose, Massachusetts, with her husband and three children.